Sugar Smart

EXPRESS

The 21-DAY Quick-Start Plan to Stop Cravings, Lose Weight, and Still Enjoy the Sweets You Love!

ANNE ALEXANDER

Editor at Large for **Prevention**® and *New York Times*
bestselling author of *The Sugar Smart Diet*

with Julia VanTine

Foreword by Holly Phillips, MD, CBS News Medical Correspondent

RODALE.

Internet addresses and telephone numbers given in this book
were accurate at the time it went to press.

© 2015 by Rodale Inc.

Photographs © 2015 by Rodale Inc.

Rodale books may be purchased for business or promotional use or for special sales. For information, please write to:
Special Markets Department, Rodale Inc., 733 Third Avenue, New York, NY 10017

Prevention is a registered trademark of Rodale Inc.

Printed in the United States of America

Rodale Inc. makes every effort to use acid-free ♾, recycled paper ♻.

Exercise photographs by Mitch Mandel. All other photos by Tom MacDonald.

Book design by Joanna Williams

Library of Congress Cataloging-in-Publication Data is on file with the publisher.

ISBN 978-1-62336-535-6 hardcover

Distributed to the trade by Macmillan

2   4   6   8   10   9   7   5   3   1   hardcover

We inspire and enable people to improve their lives and the world around them.

rodalebooks.com

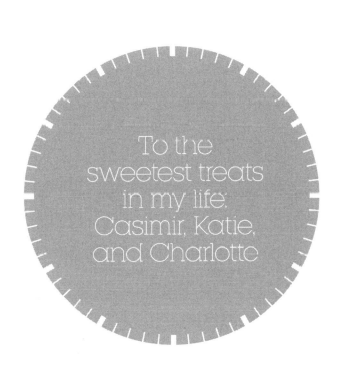

To the
sweetest treats
in my life:
Casimir, Katie,
and Charlotte

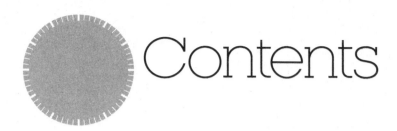

Contents

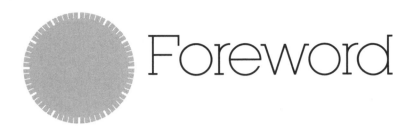# Foreword

In recent years, sugar has become ubiquitous in our culture to the point where it's practically inescapable. Of course, it's in the candy, cookies, cakes, pudding, donuts, and ice cream where we expect to see it. But these days, the sweet stuff is also showing up in foods where it really doesn't belong—including crackers, chips, pasta sauces, potato salads, breads, salad dressings, and soups—and as unsuspecting consumers, we have no idea it's there. For food manufacturers, money talks and sugar sells. Adding sugar to packaged foods makes them more appealing (and arguably addictive—but we'll get to that later) and hence makes us more likely to buy them. As a result, the food industry has essentially hijacked our taste buds, and we're craving the sweet stuff 24/7. It's a dangerous cycle: The more we crave, the more we eat, and the more we eat, the more we crave.

Anne Alexander experienced this reality firsthand shortly after she moved back to the States after spending a decade abroad. Immediately, she found her taste buds had been corrupted and her hunger had been sent into overdrive by added sugar, and she decided to figure out why. Anne's groundbreaking 2013 book, *The Sugar Smart Diet*, was the culmination of years of personal dietary detective work.

Anne was the editorial director of *Prevention* at the time, which is when I got to know her while working as a contributing editor. Anne has long been a trailblazer as a writer and editor, helping women take steps to enhance their health and their family's health: Every aspect of her work is marked by her trademark intelligence, common sense, and real-world wisdom, qualities she brings to her remarkable, engaging books. These pages truly come to life, however, because Anne is personally invested in this subject, thanks to her own (now reformed) sweet tooth.

As she uncovered in her research, Americans are OD'ing on sugar, often without realizing it, and that's a problem for our health and our waistlines. As Anne points out, the average American consumes 22 teaspoons of sugar per day (352 calories' worth!), triple the recommended limit of added sugars for a healthy diet. Excess sugar and processed foods contribute to hormonal imbalances (especially detrimental shifts in appetite-regulating hormones) and chronic, low-grade inflammation. These conditions are at the root of the most prevalent health problems in our society today—from obesity and type 2 diabetes to fatty liver disease, heart disease, and Alzheimer's disease.

In my medical practice, on a daily basis I see patients who are struggling with how to deal with sugar cravings as they try to improve their diets. Some can't give up the sugar they know they're eating—dessert and sweet treats are unbreakable habits for them—so not surprisingly, weight loss is an endlessly frustrating challenge. Meanwhile, others assume they don't consume sugar because they don't eat sweets, yet they're unaware that stealth sugars in processed foods are undoing their well-intentioned weight-loss efforts and propelling them toward myriad health problems. That's why *Sugar Smart Express* speaks to all of us.

Sugar Smart Express provides a comprehensive look at how our food supply became *sugarized* over the last 40 years, a trend that's linked directly with the obesity epidemic—as you may know, nearly two-thirds of the US population is either overweight or obese, and that number is on the rise. As Anne points out, we're physiologically programmed to like sugar, thanks to our neurologic responses to sweet tastes and the emotional pleasure we derive from consuming them. The trouble is, it's easy for this feel-good programming to spiral out of control because sugar in its many incarnations (sugars, fruit juice concentrates, syrups, honey, molasses, and anything ending in –ose, in packaged foods) stimulates our appetite. Plus, eating sugar boosts our mental and physical cravings for more, a phenomenon that researchers have called "sugar addiction"–with some even claiming that the sweet stuff is more habit-forming than cocaine.

That's where *Sugar Smart Express* comes in: In recent years, much has been written about why sugar is bad for us and how prevalent it is in our food supply. This book offers a clear path for what to do with these unfortunate realities. It provides a plan that's designed to help us retrain our taste buds to become more sensitive to sugar so that we crave less of it. Rather than advising a rigid method of eliminating sugar entirely, Anne offers a refreshingly balanced approach to becoming conscious of where it lurks in our diets and reducing our intake in manageable phases. Her goal is to help us reclaim control over the sugar we consume instead of letting stealth sources of sugar control our eating habits, our weight, our health, our moods, and more. It's about finding the sweet spot where we can consume sugar consciously, selectively, and in moderation but still maintain intentional control over how much of it we eat.

Anne's take-charge plan provides helpful strategies for how to fuel up with a high-protein breakfast (which helps curb cravings) and how to use herbs, spices, vinegars, and other ingredients to pump up the flavor of our meals without adding sugar. Her "Express Kitchen Cleanup" advice is doable and effective–as I often tell my patients, *"If it's not there, you can't eat it!"* I also love Anne's idea of creating a personal Rewards Card, a go-to cheat sheet with satisfying 20-minute pleasures you can indulge in rather than grabbing a sugary treat. This is something we should all be doing as part of good self-care, regardless of whether or not we have a demanding sweet tooth. Her shopping tips, lists of tasty ingredients to keep in the fridge and pantry, and timesaving shortcuts to help us prepare healthy meals quickly are practical and easy. Throughout the book, you'll find dozens of tempting recipes for meals and snacks.

Given our current environment, this book should be required reading for everyone who wants to lose weight, improve their health, and curb their sugar intake. Don't be surprised if you find yourself dog-earing, highlighting, or otherwise marking up the text, because these pages offer incredibly valuable strategies for reclaiming control of your eating habits and your health. As Anne writes, "It's amazing how stripping the excess sugar from your diet sweetens your life." This is true not only because doing so improves health but also because it makes sugar special again, returning it to the realm of treats where it was meant to be. That's a very sweet reality, indeed.

Holly Phillips, MD
Medical Contributor, CBS News
Author of *The Exhaustion Breakthrough*

# Introduction

Get Ready for the Sweet Life!

When I was a kid, sugar was a treat. It was dessert on Friday or Saturday nights–a piece of pie or a dish of ice cream. A Russell Stover chocolate bunny and a few Peeps on Easter morning. A single glass of Coke on Super Bowl Sunday, when my parents purchased *one* bottle, and my brothers and I got to savor that rare flavor rush. Back in the day, sugar had its time (a special occasion) and its place (on the kitchen table, in a little bowl).

Little did I know that, over the next 40 years, sugar would creep into almost every processed food on the grocery store shelf. Like most everyone else, I didn't notice this sugary invasion until I stumbled upon it with the eyes of an outsider.

Here's how my "awakening" went down. About 15 years ago, when I was an editor-in-chief at Rodale, my family and I had the chance to move first to London and, later, Eastern Europe. As the mother of three small children, I made healthy eating a priority, and it was a no-brainer in Warsaw. Fresh food markets were everywhere, and processed foods were hard to find. We ate according to the seasons and lived on real, whole food–grilled meats, fruits and locally grown veggies, thick yogurt, dense loaves of bread flecked with chunks of whole wheat and rye kernels. Ah, the bread–so chewy and filling that one slice satisfied both belly and soul.

That didn't mean we didn't love our sweets, though. On Sundays, we strolled through one of Warsaw's beautiful parks, savoring *lody*–a golf ball-size scoop of ice cream atop a waffle cone. We treasured our Sunday *lody* the same way I treasured, as a child, my sweet weekend treat.

Prompted by my desire to raise my children in America, we moved back to the States. On my first trip to the supermarket, I filled my cart with healthy choices, including whole grain cereal, whole wheat bread, and low-fat yogurt. Nothing new there–these were staples of our Eastern European diet.

What was new: my appetite. I was starving. 24/7.

In the first weeks after our arrival, we lived in a temporary apartment about 45 minutes from my kids' new school. Each morning, we shared a healthy breakfast–whole wheat toast, fruit, bran cereal or yogurt–then piled into the car. But by the time we arrived at their school, I could barely focus on kissing my kids goodbye for the day, so rumbly was my tummy. My hunger was astonishing, off the charts. I was eating my Warsaw-style breakfast every morning–what was going on?

One day, exasperated by my gnawing hunger, I drove straight back to our apartment and read the nutrition labels on my "healthy" cereal, bread, and yogurt. Every item listed sugar or high-fructose corn syrup as the second or third ingredient. I went through all of my cabinets, stocked with what I thought were healthy foods, and, damn it, sugar was everywhere: in the canned soups and chili; in the jarred pasta sauce; in the packaged noodle and rice dinners. Sugar even showed up in the whole wheat crackers we munched during the car ride home after school.

What? Having been out of the States for a decade, returning once a year for family visits, I was, in some sense, a newbie to the American diet, looking at it with fresh eyes. And the American diet ticked me off. What the hell was all of this sugar doing in my food? How was it affecting my kids' health? And how could I stop this secret glut of sugar from invading their unsuspecting little bodies?

That lightbulb moment–followed by many others–led me to conceive and write *The Sugar Smart Diet*. Published in 2013, it became a blockbuster–the revolutionary result of asking one simple question: How can we free ourselves from sugar overload and reclaim its pleasures without wrecking our health?

The answer lies in achieving what I call *sugar freedom*–breaking the powerful hold that sugar has on both body and mind. Gain sugar freedom, and yes, you'll lose weight and belly fat. But the benefits go even deeper. As the weight melts away, mood brightens, mind clears, and energy soars. This plan has helped countless people just like you to discover, and live, the sweet life. If they can do it, so can you. And now, you can do it even faster.

GOODBYE SUGAR SLAVERY, HELLO SWEET FREEDOM

The Sugar Smart Diet debuted as a *New York Times* bestseller. That was cool, to be sure. But more important to me was that the plan was changing lives. More gratifying still, I got to see those changes right before my eyes. For example, one test panelist, Robyn, lost 15 pounds and 16.5 inches on the original 32-day plan, kept going, and lost 75 more pounds! Before she got sugar smart, Robyn used a CPAP machine at night and took several prescription medications a day to treat her weight-related problems. Today? No more CPAP, and just one medication a day. (Robyn's a double winner. She road-tested this plan as well and lost nearly 12 more pounds and 13.5 more inches!)

"Now, I can feel hungry but not panicked," she says. "I have absolutely NO cravings! Food tastes so much better. I feel satisfied and full after my meals. Sugar is a drug to me, altering my perceptions about food, causing uncontrollable cravings. Without sugar, I am in control, satiated and content. I feel like I have finally unlocked the key to my success."

Sugar Smart Express shrinks the first plan to just 21 days. Why? Because the sweet life has so many perks, weight loss being just one, that I thought you'd want to start living it as soon as possible. When you understand what the sweet life entails, I think you'll want in.

When you live *la vida dulce*, you never deny yourself the pleasure of sugar. You can have chocolate. Cheesecake. Chocolate cheesecake! But you've learned not to let sugar run your show. *You* decide when, where, and how to indulge. Not your cravings. Not the doughnuts in the break room. Not the food industry. You. And while you respect sugar's power and allure, it's just one pleasure in the banquet of life.

After decades of cravings and sugar binges, I renegotiated my relationship with sugar, and today, I live the sweet life. And get this—I savor dark chocolate almost every day and devote a cabinet above my refrigerator to sugary goodies. I enjoy sugar, yet I'm free. You can be, too.

The core of sugar freedom? Making smart, informed choices. This streamlined plan gives you the knowledge you need to make those choices. You'll learn more than you ever dreamed about sugar—what forms it takes, which kinds are healthiest, and how to satisfy your natural desire for it in ways that empower you. The plan also offers you a framework for building a life of joy and satisfaction, so that you can right-size sugar's place in your diet and savor it in the ways that give you the most pleasure. The best part is, you can achieve all this in just 3 weeks' time. Skeptical? Look at the before-and-after photos in every chapter.

But before we get to the actual plan, let me tell you how it came to be.

THE DARK SIDE OF SUGAR

In 2013, I returned to Rodale to become the editorial director of *Prevention,* the top health magazine in the country. With a job like this, you read a lot of medical journals and health books and talk to a lot of experts to stay on top of hot-button public health issues. Fresh off my lightbulb moment, coming back to *Prevention* felt like fate. I set my sights on added sugars and found study after disturbing study about their impact on health.

As part of my investigation, I met with Robert Lustig, MD, of the University of California, San Francisco, whose explosive YouTube video, *Sugar: The Bitter Truth,* first sounded the alarm about added sugars and health. I'd read an early copy of his game-changing book, *Fat Chance,* and found his conclusions jaw-dropping. Talking with him about how the food industry had sugarjacked America's food choices compelled me to dig even deeper into the research. From the American Heart Association and the Centers for Disease Control to the Harvard School of Public Health, scientists are reaching consensus: The huge amount of sugar we consume, often unknowingly, is a public health crisis that can lead to obesity, type 2 diabetes, and heart disease.

Specifically, research implicates fructose, a simple sugar found naturally in fruit that's also present in refined sugars. At one time, most of the fructose in our diets came from natural foods like honey and fruit. The healthy fiber in fruit slows our bodies' absorption of fructose and acts as a natural brake on our intake of this sugar. (Can you eat 10 apples in one sitting?) But now fructose, in the form of high-fructose corn syrup, is ubiquitous in our diets. Why? As high-fructose corn syrup became cheaper to make, food manufacturers began to add it to everything—not just soda, but jarred sauces, canned soups, crackers, and prepared foods.

Even if you rarely eat sweets or drink soda, you're likely paying the price. Added sugars have seeped into virtually every food in a bottle, jar, box, or bag—and "whole grain" breakfast cereals and "100 percent whole wheat" breads aren't the solution. Yes, these foods contain whole wheat or whole grains. But they're *highly processed* whole wheat or whole grains. And during processing, their fiber—the stuff that slows digestion—is pulverized. What was healthy, digestion-slowing roughage is ground into powder, puffed, or flaked. As far as your body is concerned, highly refined whole grain crackers or fluffy whole wheat bread isn't much more nutritious than a Pop-Tart. (Of course, portion sizes matter, too.)

To add insult to injury, added sugars seem to supercharge our appetites. In a study published in the *Journal of the American Medical Association,* researchers looked at brain-imaging scans after people consumed fructose or another simple sugar called glucose. Fructose altered bloodflow in areas of the brain that stimulate appetite, the study found; glucose did not. What this means is that eating refined sugars may trigger cravings for more of the stuff that thickens our waists and threatens our health! No wonder I had such intense cravings when I moved back to the States. My brain was being flooded by the sudden surge of refined sugar.

SUGAR FREEDOM, HERE WE COME!

As I pored over the research, sugar became an obsession. At the supermarket, I'd pick up items at random, read their Nutrition Facts labels, and gasp out loud. Seriously? Thirty-three grams of sugar in a cup of yogurt? Twenty-five grams in a frozen entrée? Ten grams in those kid-friendly tubes of yogurt? That's 2½ teaspoons of sugar, in one 2-ounce tube! I used to feel good about tucking them into my kids' lunch boxes! Oh, I was fuming.

Deep in my sugar-outrage stage, I unthinkingly bought potato salad from the deli section of my supermarket for a party. I opened the lid, sampled a forkful, and–*geez!* Even my kids, who love their cookies and ice cream, thought it was sickeningly sweet. What is sugar doing in potato salad?

There's this feeling I get when I know I have to write a book. That no-turning-back moment was sealed after I met with my longtime colleague and *Prevention* advisor Andrew Weil, MD. I asked him what one change he would recommend to *Prevention* readers that could dramatically reduce their risk of chronic disease.

"Cut out sugar-sweetened drinks," he replied.

I nodded my agreement. I'd read the studies linking sweetened drinks with obesity, diabetes, and heart disease. But then I thought, *What about people who don't drink sugary drinks–who think they're eating healthy? What can they do to break free from the insane amounts of sugar in processed food?*

I decided to devise a plan that would break sugar's powerful grip on our bodies and minds and put us back in charge of our weight and health. I didn't want to demonize sugar. (You'll have to pry my peanut-butter ice cream from my cold, dead hands!) I wanted to *reclaim* it. I envisioned a plan that would steer our inborn desire for sugar back to healthy, natural sources of sweetness and teach us how to savor sugar *when and how we consciously chose to,* rather than cave into out-of-control cravings.

Fired up, I welcomed the challenge. I felt like Mel Gibson in *Braveheart:* They can spike our potato salad with high-fructose corn syrup, but they can't take our sugar freedom!

THEY CAME, THEY ATE, THEY LOST WEIGHT

One of the best things about the Sugar Smart diet is that it's been road-tested–twice. In the original plan, our test panel dropped up to 16 pounds and 16 inches in 32 days. On this express version, our panel lost an average of 7 pounds and 7 inches in 21 days, with some panelists losing up to 15 pounds and 14 inches. Sweet success!

Of course, the primary reason for this success is replacing processed fare with whole foods, which automatically limits added sugars. But I think a huge, secondary one is because the food is so unbelievably good. I insisted that this meal plan be just as tasty as the original. My crack team of registered dietitians delivered, with our panelists giving the thumbs up or thumbs-down.

When I renegotiated my relationship with sugar, I learned that there's a huge difference between both flavor and sweetness, and between natural and artificial sweetness. Our panelists–both sets–learned that, and you will, too. Once the plan "reboots" your taste buds, you'll detect the natural sweetness in whole foods, from crunchy broccoli to thick, delicious plain yogurt. When chocolate reappears on the menu, you'll be in sugar heaven. (Yes, you get chocolate on this plan!)

The effectiveness of the Sugar Smart Diet–including this streamlined version–lies in its unique, three-pronged approach to sugar.

It addresses your body's physiological "pull" toward sugar as well as the powerful emotional connection that many people experience. Built around nutritious whole foods, our meals and snacks short-circuit cravings–and satisfy hunger and our inborn desire for sweetness–by bringing levels of hormones that drive hunger, fullness, and cravings into harmony. (Before the sugarjacking of our food supply, they harmonized a lot better.)

If you tend to soothe stress or negative emotions with food, the emotional coping strategies in every chapter will give you positive alternatives to "cookie therapy." Unlike a fistful of Chips Ahoy!–a temporary fix, at best–these techniques offer the lasting comfort, calm, and sense of control you seek.

I can vouch for this. In college, stressed by exams and looking to fuel all-night study sessions, I turned to doughnuts and Snickers bars for quick energy. It took me a while, but eventually I noticed that these sugar rushes were quickly followed by sugar binges. Fortunately, I learned to recognize when sugar cravings are building, and how to short-circuit a potential sugar binge. You will, too.

It reduces intake of added sugars automatically and deliciously. Our plan slashes the Straight-Up Sugars in sweets and sodas as well as the Secret Sugars that lurk in foods you'd never think of. But you're not likely to miss them for long–the all-new menu is just as fabulous as the original. Linda, who lost 15 pounds on the Express Plan, says the Strawberry No-Bake Cheesecake Parfait (see page 209) is "simple and delicious." Alison, who lost 11 pounds, pronounces the California Roast Beef Pita Sandwich (see page 168) "quick and delicious." (Quick, simple, delicious–definitely words you want to hear when you're following a weight-loss plan.)

It sets its sights on Sugar Mimics. I've already mentioned the pitfalls of refined carbs and highly processed whole grain products. On this plan, you'll dramatically reduce your intake of both, swapping them for healthier alternatives that taste just as good.

In short, you'll reap benefits sweeter than a handful of gummy bears. By cutting added sugars and adding pleasure to every day, the Express Plan will help you:

- Crush cravings for sugar and carbs
- Lose weight
- Flatten a sugar belly
- Flip the switch from tired out to fired up
- Cut your risk of diabetes, heart disease, and other chronic diseases
- Enjoy sugary treats when you choose to, not because you need to

The cherry on top? Personal advice and tips from *Prevention* advisors, including Dr. Andrew Weil, Dr. Arthur Agatston, and Dr. David Katz, along with pros like Dr. Pamela Peeke and Ashley Koff, RD. It's comforting to know that even the experts struggle with sugar cravings–and even better when they tell you how to shut 'em down.

THE PERKS AND PROMISES OF THE SWEET LIFE

One of my heroes is Mohandas Gandhi, whose nonviolent approach to tyranny inspired a nation and changed the world. Something he said has always inspired me: "Happiness is when what you think, what you say, and what you do are in harmony." We can take a similar approach to changing our relationship with sugar. Specifically, we can align our new knowledge about sugar with making conscious choices to consume it in a way that makes us happy.

When you gain new information, as you will in these pages, you have your own lightbulb moment. The negative chatter in your head that stops you from giving your diet, health, and life the care they deserve is silenced. A new, empowering inner voice emerges. And when that happens, you begin to treat your body and your soul with the same nurturing care that you lavish on those you love. It's pretty simple: When you know better, you do better and feel better about everything in your life, not just your diet.

We've all swan-dived into sugar to cool stress or hide from feelings or situations we'd rather not deal with. But on this plan, the only good reason to eat sugar is a positive one–to gift our tongues and (as you'll learn) our brains with its pleasures. Stick to that one reason, and sugar returns to its proper place in your diet: as a treat to be savored with eyes-closed bliss.

It's amazing how stripping the excess sugar from your diet sweetens your life. On this plan, you'll ask yourself questions like, How can I nurture myself right now? Do I "need" this chocolate, or is a hug, a long walk, or a shoulder to cry on what I'm craving? What did I do today just for fun? What choices can I make today that will empower and revitalize me?

One of the best things about the plan (besides the weight loss, of course) is that it makes sugar special again. After periods of eating it mindlessly, not really tasting those doughnuts and candy bars, I came full circle to my experience of sugar as a kid: It's a treat again. But so is stargazing on a summer night, or getting on a toboggan with your kids for the first time in years, or choosing to spend a rare free hour getting a pedicure rather than paying bills online because pretty toes make you feel good.

My point: In this food-centric society, we rarely deprive ourselves of food. It's plentiful, quick, and often cheap. It's the other, more deeply satisfying pleasures that we cut out because we are too busy. I think we have it backward. This plan will change your weight, no question. The proof is in those before-and-after photos. But if you let it, it might also change your life.

We'll talk more about the perks of putting yourself first later in the book. Before I do that, I want to tell you about the "sugarizing" of our food supply for the past 40 years. You may be shocked or even angry. But at long last, you'll learn the truth about the rising tide of added sugars in our diet–implicated in obesity and chronic disease–and get a glimpse of the solution that will lead you to the sweet life.

The Sugarjacking of America

Centuries ago, sugar–the real deal, straight from the cane–was as rare and precious as gold. Today, we live in a Willy Wonka wonderland. Gummy bears! Doughnuts! Sweet tea! Chocolate! What's a birthday without cake? A holiday minus the cookies? A summer night *sans* ice cream? At the banquet of life, sweets rule supreme. Anytime we celebrate family, tradition, life's transitions–life itself–there's sugar, smack in the middle of all that love and joy and good cheer.

But there's a catch. The more sugar we eat, the more we want. And the fatter and sicker we get as a nation.

Another day, another study that suggests a link between diets high in added sugar and increased risk of diseases of civilization. Obesity. Type 2 diabetes. Cardiovascular disease. Cancer. Meanwhile, too many Americans feel chained to their desire for sugar or don't even realize they're bound. Their shackles: extra pounds.

We Americans are big on taking personal responsibility for our health.

We take our vitamins, eat our veggies, suck it up and get our mammograms and prostate exams. While it's true that we love our sweets, our sugary dilemma is not entirely of our own making.

In the past 40 years, ever-increasing amounts of sugar have invaded the American diet. We consume far more than we realize, in foods we never suspect. Each year, assuming you're on par with the average American, you swallow 78 pounds of added sugars–that is, sugar that's an ingredient in food rather than sugar that's naturally occurring in food. That 78 pounds equates to almost sixteen 5-pound bags! Manufacturers may add processed sugars (such as cane sugar or high-fructose corn syrup, or HFCS), natural sugars (such as fructose), or both to all sorts of common foods.

The food industry has dealt us a double whammy. First, it's hijacked our natural, inborn attraction to sugar–give most of us a choice between an apple and a doughnut, and there's typically no contest. Second, food manufacturers have sugarjacked the food supply, adding sweeteners to virtually every processed edible. It's one thing to *know* you're eating sugary treats. It's quite another to discover that staples like bread, deli meats, and canned soups are laced with the stuff.

Added sugars aren't the only issue. We're also drowning in refined carbohydrates. Refined carbs typically contain both the processed sugars listed above *and* white flour and/or processed whole grains, which break down and are digested as rapidly as sugar. In other words, these "junk carbs" behave like sugar in your body. (More about refined carbs in Chapter 2.)

As you may suspect by now, there's a dark side to Wonkaville. But there's light at the end of the tunnel. You're about to acquire *sugar smarts*–the knowledge you need to outwit the food industry's tricks and enjoy your favorite sugary indulgences in a healthy, balanced way. Gaining sugar smarts pays off big, and more quickly than you might think. By the end of the Sugar Smart Express Plan, you'll be slimmer, more energized, and fueled to be your best self, body and soul. But before we go there, let me explain how we arrived at this sugar-drenched state of affairs.

ANATOMY OF A SUGARJACKING

In 1978, while I was feathering my hair like Jaclyn Smith in *Charlie's Angels,* 13 percent of men and 17 percent of women were obese (meaning they had a BMI greater than 30).

By the late 1980s, those rates had risen to 18 and 25 percent, respectively.

In 2001, Americans first heard the phrase "obesity epidemic."

By 2003, a shocking 32 percent of men and 35 percent of women were obese.

Whoa. In 25 years, obesity rates in America more than doubled. Rates of type 2 diabetes and metabolic syndrome—both associated with obesity—had skyrocketed, too (see page 29).

What happened? Obesity is complicated. You can't point a finger at any one cause. But it's worth noting that two significant changes in the American diet occurred during that 25-year period.

The first change: the rise of the low-fat diet. In 1977, 3 years before the introduction of the Dietary Guidelines for Americans, a Senate report recommended that we reduce our intake of dietary fat. We listened, drastically cutting back on even those fats that current research shows are healthy.

In response to our fat phobia, the food industry swung into action, rolling out fat-free everything—chips, ice cream, granola bars, muffins. SnackWell's cookies were born, with just as many empty calories but zero fat. (Of course I bought them. I could eat cookies? And not get fat? Ah, the wonders of science!) Even manufacturers of cereals, bagels, and pasta—which are naturally low in fat—slapped "naturally fat-free" on their labels. By the mid-1990s, SnackWell's Madness was in full swing. The number of new reduced- or low-fat products rose steeply, reaching 2,076 in 1996 before sinking to 481 in 1999.

These products may have contained little or no fat, but many did contain sugar. Lots of it. (And those that didn't contain sugar were comprised primarily of white flour.)

And that was the second major dietary change: HFCS became the nation's primary caloric sweetener. Between 1970 and 1990, its use skyrocketed 1,000 percent. (That's no typo. *One thousand percent*.)

By the end of the 1980s, HFCS had replaced cane sugar in sodas; food manufacturers followed suit soon after. That's why the earliest research on the potential link between obesity and HFCS focused on soft drink consumption.

SnackWell's Madness hit the ash can of fad-diet history a long time ago. We've made peace with heart-healthy fats like olive oil, nuts and seeds, and avocado. But the added sugars that gave low-fat and fat-free foods their appeal remain in virtually all processed foods, and our consumption of added sugars, particularly fructose, has doubled in the past 30 years.

The Top Three Reasons We Snarf So Much Sugar

Well, yes, it tastes divine—no argument there! But probe a bit deeper, and there are three main factors that affect our intake of added sugars.

- **The we're-only-human factor.** Our bodies have a normal, inborn attraction to sugar—it's part of our hardware. Some of us have an emotional connection to sugar as well, often forged early in life.
- **The who-woulda-thunk-it factor.** If your diet is packed with quick-and-easy processed foods—frozen lasagna and breakfast sandwiches, "all-natural" whole grain cereals or granola bars, jarred sauces of all kinds—you might be amazed to learn how much sugar they're packing. Even if you read the ingredients lists, you may not recognize sugar's many aliases. (You'll find 39 of them on page 18.)
- **The but-it-doesn't-taste-sweet factor.** From white bread to white rice, spaghetti to saltines, refined carbs may not always have a sugary taste, but they act like sugar in the body, fueling cravings for sweets and more refined carbs.

THE RISE OF THE SUGAR BELLY

This insidious national slide toward added sugars may be affecting you right now. If you find that your mood and energy levels are crashing as your weight is rising, a sugar- and carb-drenched diet may be the culprit. And that's even if you think you're choosing good-for-you foods. In fact, without knowing it, you may be experiencing the consequences of added-sugar overload right now.

Do you . . .

- Feel famished an hour after your morning fruit-flavored yogurt, energy bar, or "healthy" fruit smoothie from the coffee shop?
- Avoid soda and sweets and choose whole grain bread and cereal, but struggle with fatigue and sugar cravings?
- Fight valiantly against helping yourself to treats at work, only to cave in when you're nodding off at your desk?
- Reward yourself with comfort food after a brutal day or when you feel low?
- Keep the top button of your jeans undone most days because you've gained weight and your belly is getting bigger?

These are all signs of a physical and emotional tie to the added sugars in processed foods and drinks that, over time, can lead to a big gain in body fat, especially around your middle. This is what I call a sugar belly, and it can cause more than just a bad day in the department store dressing room. There's mounting evidence that consuming too much of one type of sugar—in particular, fructose—is a major player in the epidemic-level rates of obesity and diabetes. Fructose causes you to pack on fat and may bypass many of the body's "I'm full" signals, which may promote overeating, weight gain, and insulin resistance, a body chemistry glitch considered a risk factor for diabetes and heart disease.

"Well, okay," you say, "but my belly is just fine, thank you. What I'm doing must be working." Not so fast. If your diet is mostly fast-food fare and frothy coffee concoctions topped with towers of whipped cream, you may be packing on fat where you can't see it: in your liver. Even if you're rocking skinny jeans and appear to be otherwise healthy. As you'll see in Chapter 3, a fatty liver may tip the body into metabolic disarray and disease.

But we have sweet news: You can shrink your sugar belly without swearing off sugar forever. Talk about having your cake and eating it, too! Jumping off where our best-selling book, *The Sugar Smart Diet*, ended, the Express Plan helps you take control of your sugar intake, outsmart hidden sugars, lose weight, protect your health, and enjoy one of nature's greatest treats on *your* terms and in less time.

Even Cavemen Loved the Sweet Stuff

Nuts and berries or Chips Ahoy!? Odds are, our caveman forebears would have picked the cookies. Early humans associated a sweet taste with calorie-dense foods such as fruit, experts believe. With their entire existence focused on getting enough to eat, every calorie counted, and sweetness meant "food" and "safe."

For a while, calorie-dense fruit and honey were virtually all we knew of sweet. In the Paleolithic era, a period of half a million years that ended around 10,000 years ago, fruits and veggies made up an estimated 65 percent of humans' diet. Things started to change with the birth of agriculture. Humans began to rely on cereal grains, and fruit and veggie consumption dropped to 20 percent or less. And sugar—derived from sugarcane and cultivated in tiny amounts at first—began its delicious, relentless seduction.

Our bodies were designed to crave sugar, store it easily, and use it fast. But we live in high-tech times, and while we're still hardwired to seek sugar, we store more than we use. And we're not climbing trees to pluck fruit, either. We're hitting drive-thrus and calling for free delivery.

Never fear. The Express Plan works with your body's natural attraction to sugar and is packed with the vitamins, minerals, and other nutrients your body needs. As you'll discover, something as simple as eating a high-protein breakfast helps rein in your appetite during the day and reduces snacking on high-sugar foods at night.

Short and sweet—that's the Express approach. First, you *reduce* the amount of sugar you eat, which retrains your taste buds and eating habits. Then, you *reclaim* sugar, returning it to your diet in a healthful way. You learn how much added sugar you should eat on a typical day, when it's appropriate to indulge in a little extra, and the right ways to enjoy a sweet treat. In just 21 days, you're on the path to sugar freedom.

SLIM DOWN, FEEL GREAT: RESETTING YOUR "SUGAR THERMOSTAT"

Countless couples have waged the War of the Thermostat. He likes the house toasty. She prefers Arctic-like temperatures. (Or vice versa.) In that situation, there's just one way to make peace: agree to keep the thermostat midway between Mediterranean heat and Siberian cold.

On this plan, you'll find your sugar midpoint. At this "sweet spot," your attraction to sugar isn't so hot that it contributes to weight gain and unhealthy belly fat, or so cold that you feel deprived of your favorite treats. In fact, identifying that midpoint frees you to enjoy those foods every day, if you wish—for the right reasons, and in the proper amounts.

Resetting your sugar thermostat helps you achieve sugar freedom in two ways: **It dials down your body's physical attraction to sugar and cools your emotional connection with it.** On this plan, you reduce your sugar intake in stages and then cut it out completely for less than a week as you learn practical tools that temper sugar withdrawal and replace the reward of a sugar rush with healthier pleasures. This strategy resets your taste buds. Once you reintroduce sugar into your diet, it will taste intensely sweet, and you'll be satisfied with less (way less).

It sets the stage for metabolic harmony. Dramatically curtailing your sugar consumption also resets your metabolism. Your insulin levels will fall, and your body's ability to burn fat will improve. Levels of the hunger hormone ghrelin will drop, and your body's response to the appetite-quelling hormone, leptin, will improve. As insulin, ghrelin, and leptin once again work in concert to manage hunger and cravings, metabolic harmony is achieved, the sugar belly flattens, and the risk of disease falls. (We'll explain exactly how these hormones can go awry and affect your appetite and cravings in the next chapter.)

Once you begin to introduce sugars back into your diet, you'll add them slowly and in a particular way, so you can determine how you feel without all that sugar in your system. I think you'll feel awesome. Your cravings will be history. You'll have traded in those sugar rushes and crashes for the steady energy provided by clean eating and nonfood rewards. And, of course, your jeans will fit the way they used to.

Sugar's Emotional Hooks

While our taste buds and brains crave the delightful reward of sugar, so do our hearts. Who among us hasn't turned to craptastic sweets and junk food to get the comforting warm fuzzies we need when we're emotionally wrung out? It's not really the sugar we crave, but the relief it seems to deliver—one sweet, gooey, soothing mouthful at a time.

But more often than not, sugar's promise of comfort is an empty one, especially when we eat to soothe troubling emotions such as anxiety, loneliness, anger, or boredom. That's called emotional eating, and let me tell you, it's real. According to therapists who specialize in treating emotional eating, one sign of using sugar to manage emotions is that responding to a sugar craving—eating, say, chocolate or ice cream to satisfy it—doesn't alleviate it. Rather, trying to satisfy the craving prompts a desire for more.

Memory plays a key role in the link between sugar and feelings. Many of the sugary foods we love and crave transport us back to times when we felt loved and cared for. Habit ties into the emotional attraction, too. If you're used to having a doughnut for breakfast, cookies in the afternoon, or dessert after dinner, something feels off if you skip it.

Do you feel "hooked"? If so, exploring your relationship with sugar—as you will in the Express Countdown (Chapter 6)—can help you untangle the feelings and patterns that draw you to sugary, fatty foods.

THE SUGAR SMART EXPRESS PLAN

Sometimes, a month is just too long to wait for good things to happen. So although you know it's not healthy, you try yet another crash or fad diet. The Sugar Smart Express Plan is different. It teams the nutritious eating plan you need for good health, lasting energy, and a healthy weight with the quick results you want. Centered on whole foods, this plan weans you off added sugars and satisfies with lean protein, whole grains (*real* whole grains), veggies, fruit, and lots and lots of flavor. Once the weight starts to come off and your sweet tooth is tamed, sugar is reintroduced in a balanced way. Take a look at what's ahead.

Days 1 to 3: The Express Countdown

I have to confess, the cold-turkey method of quitting anything, sugar included, doesn't appeal to me. Too much of a shock to the system. So the Countdown is perfect for chickens like me (and you might appreciate it, too). As you follow your regular diet, you'll assess how much added sugar you're currently consuming and reduce your intake step by step. In just 72 hours, you'll have begun to break your physiological and emotional connection to sugar and reduce sugar overload's harmful effects.

Days 4 to 7: Phase 1: Escape from Sugarville

Here's where the Express Plan really ramps up! For 4 days, you'll eliminate all sugar from your diet (even fruit), as well as all products made from processed grain, whether refined or whole. Okay, it's a challenge, although many of our test panelists did just fine. But you'll love the results: By the end of Day 7, our test panelists lost an average of 4 pounds. Plus, this phase introduces simple strategies that ease sugar withdrawal and replace the reward of a sugar rush with healthier routes to pleasure. The tasty, satisfying meals we've provided will help, too.

Days 8 to 11: Phase 2: Fruitylicious!

Fruit is back, and now that you've reset your sugar thermostat, it will taste sweeter and more satisfying than ever before. The best part: You get to splurge on your favorite fruits–plump, juicy berries, exotic tropical fruit, whatever you desire. If you're an unrepentant carb-lover, rejoice. Starting in this phase, you'll enjoy a daily serving of a low-sugar whole grain bread product as well.

Days 12 to 16: Phase 3: Sugar, Naturally

To help make whole foods even more enjoyable, this phase reintroduces some straight-from-nature sweeteners, including honey, dried fruit, and maple syrup. We chose them because they have some nutritional value and are actually sweeter than cane sugar, so you don't need to use as much of them. Whole grain pasta and bread are also included; you can continue to have them once a day.

Days 17 to 21: Phase 4: The Sweet Life

Want a cookie? You can have one. In this phase, you'll learn how sweet life can be on 6 to 9 teaspoons of added sugar a day. Each day, you can have fruit, one serving of a natural sweetener from Phase 3, plus a daily serving of a processed whole grain product–regular or whole wheat. And we have some delicious treats in store for you, none containing more than 3 teaspoons of added sugar.

OPTIONAL: THE EXPRESS WORKOUT

If you're already exercising, stick with what you're doing! If not, a daily brisk walk may help speed up your weight loss. Consider doing our Express

Workout (see page 245), too. It's mini, but mighty: Four moves, three times a week, can help preserve the calorie-burning muscle you currently have. And the more muscle you have, the better equipped your body is to process sugar and carbs. As a bonus, a walk and the workout can help brighten your mood and manage stress. That's important if you make a beeline to sweets when you're frazzled.

Ready for your first shot of sugar smarts? In the next chapter, you'll get familiar with the three main types of sugar in the processed fare you eat and drink. Because the stuff in your sugar bowl isn't the only kind you're putting in your body.

Added Sugars:
A Triple Threat

For 10 seconds, forget about your weight, the ice cream in the freezer, every talk-show segment or Internet headline you've caught about sugar and health. Drag everything you think you know about the sweet stuff to your mental recycle bin and hit Delete.

Now, consider your flower or vegetable garden, or the prettiest tree in your backyard, or the plant on your sunniest windowsill. Sugar helps it grow. Sugar keeps it alive.

All green plants are sugar factories. Using the sun's energy and the green pigment in plants called chlorophyll (in a process called photosynthesis), plants convert carbon dioxide and water into oxygen and *glucose*, the basic sugar molecule from which all carbohydrates (sugars, starches, and fiber) are made.

Sugar keeps you alive, too. Glucose in your bloodstream, called blood sugar, is the fuel your body runs on (sorry, Dunkin' Donuts). Glucose is made from any carbohydrate that passes your lips, whether you're savoring chocolate truffles or wild ones.

In the broadest sense of the word, sugar is life. There's the sugar your body, and most life-forms, runs on. There's the naturally occurring sugar in the plants we eat. And then there are the refined sugars added to virtually every processed food, from the obvious (marshmallow Peeps) to the odd (beef jerky).

The Express Plan categorizes added sugars into three main types–a sugar triple threat, if you will. Consider this chapter your formal introduction. First, we'll explore dietary sugar itself: its chemical makeup and its relation to carbohydrates. Then we'll get to the "types"–what they are and the foods and beverages in which they typically lurk.

SUGAR 101

Any discussion about dietary sugar begins with carbohydrates–"saccharides," chemists call them. Sugars are the building blocks of all carbs, whether they take the form of barley or Ben & Jerry's. To get a handle on sugar's chemical structure, imagine those big, colorful, plastic Snap-Lock Beads babies play with.

In your mind, hold one green bead. That's glucose, found naturally in honey, maple syrup, and other naturally occurring foods. Glucose is the primary form of energy for the muscles and the brain.

Pick up a pink bead. That's fructose, the sugar found naturally in fruit.

There's one more sugar, galactose, found only in milk. Make that one a blue bead.

Glucose, fructose, and galactose are monosaccharides, consisting of one molecule of sugar. Eventually, any type of sugar or starch that passes your lips ends up as a monosaccharide in your body. As you'll learn, glucose and fructose are the ones that have the greatest impact on your weight and health.

Now, pop two of those beads together. Bingo–you've made a disaccharide, a sugar comprised of two molecules of sugar.

Snap the green and pink beads together. One molecule of glucose plus one molecule of fructose add up to sucrose–plain old white table sugar, derived from sugar beets or sugarcane.

Join the green and blue beads (glucose plus galactose), and you've got lactose, the sugar in milk.

Connect two green beads together, and you get maltose, the sugar that results from the fermentation of the starch in grains (such as in making bread or brewing beer).

That's where the bead game ends. You don't have the time, or beads, to model the sugars in complex carbs, which are long chains of hundreds or even thousands of glucose molecules. These polysaccharides put the *complex* in complex carbohydrates. There are two basic types of polysaccharides in plant foods: starch and fiber. Starch is found in corn, legumes such as peas and beans, grains, and tubers like potatoes. Fiber, found in varying amounts in plant foods, passes through our stomach and intestines largely undigested. But don't think it's useless—fiber helps you feel full, slows the breakdown of sugars and starches, and helps feed the trillions of friendly bacteria that promote a healthy gut, which itself plays a key role in your mood, energy level, and perhaps even your weight.

And there you have it. In general, simple carbohydrates = simple sugars, whether derived from fruit salad or Skittles. Complex carbohydrates from starchy veggies and whole grains = complex chains of glucose molecules "packaged" in fiber, nutrients, and health-promoting plant chemicals.

Now, make a further distinction between the sugars found in nature and those refined and added by man. The former are found in yogurt and apples and honey and quinoa. The latter show up in foods and beverages dreamed up by marketing departments and manufactured in industrial parks. A simple distinction, yes. But it's the cornerstone of sugar smarts.

Joelle Junior

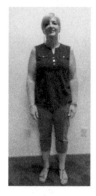

As a health editor and walking coach, Joelle Junior was skeptical of extreme or fad diets or programs that cut out certain types of foods, despite hearing friends and colleagues sing the praises of going sugar free. Her motto was "everything in moderation." But despite eating relatively healthfully, hitting the gym regularly, and walking half-marathons, she'd been stuck on a plateau for more than 6 months and couldn't budge those last 10 pounds.

"Moderation wasn't working," she explains. "I needed a kick start to get off the plateau."

When Joelle started the Sugar Smart Express Plan, she discovered that she could survive without Diet Coke and could pass up doughnuts, M&Ms, and an assortment of other goodies during her office's Chocolate Fridays. Her addiction was to the Sugar Mimics—rolls, pizza, bread, and cereal. "Even though I ate so-called healthier cereals, like plain or Multi Grain Cheerios, or various Kashi cereals, I was still getting lots of sugar because I'd have cereal 5 days out of 7."

It was that addiction that caused Joelle, who had lost nearly 9 pounds after Phase 1, to slip on the final weekend of the 21-day program. That weekend, Joelle and her husband completed the last two legs of their summer adventure to bicycle the entire New Jersey shoreline. "I was riding 60 to 70 miles, and I felt like I had a little leeway to cheat," says Joelle. "I had been dying for pizza." Along with the pizza over the 2 days, Joelle had a Diet Coke, a small ice cream cone, two fried green tomatoes with marinara, a sandwich on white bread, and a few french fries. "I had this delusion that biking all day would balance it out, but I felt bloated, weighed down, and backed up." The result: a 5-pound gain from Friday to Monday.

"It was very eye-opening," she says. "I had no idea how badly refined carbs disagree with me and make it harder for me to lose weight. And the things I craved didn't even live up to the expectation."

While Joelle slipped, she didn't fall. Monday after her weigh-in she was back on track. When she returned 2 weeks later, the 5 pounds that had crept on were gone and she lost a few more, for a total weight loss of 11.3 pounds. Plus, she shrank a total of 6 inches. The slipup weekend cemented for Joelle how well the program works: "Lesson learned!"

5.3
POUNDS LOST

AGE:
45
ALL-OVER INCHES LOST:
2.5
SUGAR SMART WISDOM:
"Foods you used to crave won't live up to the anticipation when you try them again."

STEALTH SUGARS:
NOW YOU SEE 'EM, NOW YOU DON'T

Set down the "whole grain" cereal. Back away from those "healthy" energy bars. I'm about to lay down the Two Rules of Sugar Club.

1. If it comes in a box, bag, wrapper, or can, it's a sugar bomb until you've proven it otherwise.
2. There are two main types of added sugars in foods: the kind you know about and the kind you don't.

Straight-Up Sugar

Found in candy, sweetened soft drinks (sodas, juice drinks, flavored milks, coffee drinks), sweetened breakfast cereals, energy and cereal bars, and desserts, this type of sugar is right out there, loud and proud. While it's often listed as "sugar" on a food's ingredient label, it might also be called by any number of different names, such as:

Agave nectar	Corn sweetener
Barley malt	Corn syrup
Beet sugar	Corn syrup solids
Brown rice syrup	Crystalline fructose
Brown sugar	Date sugar
Buttered sugar	Dextrose
Cane crystals	Evaporated cane juice
Cane juice	Fructose
Cane sugar	Fruit juice concentrates
Caramel	Glucose
Carob syrup	High-fructose corn syrup
Castor sugar	Honey
Coconut sugar	Invert sugar

Lactose	Rice syrup
Maltose	Sorghum
Malt syrup	Sorghum syrup
Molasses	Sucrose
Muscovado sugar	Syrup
Raw sugar	Turbinado sugar
Rice bran syrup	

Many of these sugars were a mystery to me, so I looked them up. For the record, "sorghum" is a grain best known for its end product: sweet sorghum syrup. In fact, the plant is called sorghum cane. Muscovado sugar is very dark brown—the color of cinnamon—with a strong molasses flavor. Crystalline fructose, which sounds positively trippy, is typically produced from fructose-enriched corn syrup. It's a dry powder used mostly in sweetened beverages. The stuff in that little bowl on your table is just the tip of a massive sugary iceberg.

If you haven't been reading a food's list of ingredients before you toss it into your shopping cart, now's the time to start! It's the only fail-safe way to ferret out added sugars in packaged and processed foods. Don't worry about memorizing the list. You'll see it again—and make use of it—in Chapter 6.

Secret Sugar

When it comes to food selection and abundance, Americans are the luckiest shoppers on Earth. In 1975, there were roughly 9,000 products in the average supermarket, according to the Food Marketing Institute. By 2008, there were almost 44,000! Of course, some are nonfood items—toothpaste, pot holders, that sort of thing. But there's no denying that the food selection we enjoy is mind-boggling. Which is why it's so frustrating that the majority of the packaged and processed foods we're free to choose are laced with some form of added sugar.

That's where that "cheat sheet" we just discussed and that you'll be

High-Fructose Corn Syrup:
It's All Goo

Added to a myriad of products from beverages to bread—even whole grain varieties—high-fructose corn syrup (HFCS) is the Kim Kardashian of processed food: You can't get away from it.

Forty years ago, most foods in the United States were sweetened with cane sugar. But in the 1970s, Japanese researchers discovered how to convert cornstarch into a substance sweet enough to replace the pricier cane sugar. That substance: HFCS, which bears only a passing resemblance to actual corn syrup, the thick, clear bottled liquid in the baking aisle of your supermarket.

Corn syrup proper is cornstarch that has been broken down into individual glucose molecules; it is essentially 100 percent glucose. To make HFCS, enzymes are added to corn syrup to convert some of the glucose to fructose. The result: corn syrup on steroids. It's not just sweet. It's aggressively sweet. And compared to the pure glucose in corn syrup, HFCS is high in fructose. While the body can process the small amounts of fructose found in natural foods such as fruit, it was never designed to handle the glut of fructose we consume in processed foods today.

In 1979, a paper published in an obscure journal devoted to California agriculture made a prediction that would have whizzed over the head of everyone but a handful of researchers and the food industry. Today, the paper's title gives it away: "High Fructose Corn Syrup: An Important New Sugar Substitute." And the prediction was: "Adoption of HFCS is projected to be rapid between 1978 and 1984 and would be essentially completed by 1990." As it turned out, a 1990 Yale study conducted on 14 healthy kids found that those who ate the sugar equivalent of two frosted cupcakes a day had a tenfold increase in adrenaline and exhibited abnormal behavior. People began cutting their intake of cane sugar. That's when food companies pulled a switcheroo, using less sugar and more HFCS.

Food manufacturers make different formulations of HFCS. The most common forms contain either 42 percent or 55 percent fructose. HFCS 42 is mainly used in processed foods, cereals, baked goods, and some beverages, while HFCS 55 is used primarily in soft drinks. Food manufacturers use HFCS for several reasons. It improves the consistency of processed foods and extends shelf life. It also makes sweet foods cheaper—good for food manufacturers, but not so good for you! As you'll see, the large amount of fructose we're consuming—much of it in the form of HFCS—is being implicated as a primary factor in overweight and chronic disease.

invited to use during the Sugar Smart Express Countdown will come in handy. Wander down any center aisle of your supermarket. Pick up bottles, jars, and boxes at random. More often than not, you're likely to find one of sugar's many aliases listed as an ingredient. For example, one serving of a popular canned tomato soup packs 3 teaspoons of sugar (in the form of high-fructose corn syrup) per serving. But who eats just $1/2$ cup? You eat the whole can, right? And when you do, you're swallowing $7^{1}/_{2}$ teaspoons!

True to their name, however, Secret Sugars lurk in foods you don't even think of as sweet. These include:

Pasta sauce	Cooking sauces and marinades
Canned soups	Ketchup
Frozen entrées (low calorie or otherwise)	Barbecue sauce
Salad dressings	Some processed meats (lunchmeat, hot dogs, bacon, breakfast sausages)
Dips and spreads	

There are also sweeteners that you may not realize are sugar. For example, despite its natural-sounding name, agave nectar contains more fructose than table sugar does. And a popular brand of yogurt came under legal fire in 2012 for its simultaneous use of evaporated cane juice and claim of "no sugar added." (A brief aside: As you'll learn below, artificial sweeteners are problematic for several reasons and aren't allowed on this plan.) Fortunately, you'll have your cheat sheet of added sugars to help you navigate the supermarket aisles. Once you're familiar with the many names for sugar that appear in a product's ingredients list, you'll be better prepared to control your sugar choices.

However, there's yet another group of foods that wreaks havoc on your weight and health. Technically, they're not sugars, but they may as well be because they act like sugar in your body. And chances are, they are in your kitchen and pantry right now.

Why the Sugar Smart Express Plan Shuns Sugar Substitutes

If you're a fan of diet drinks and sugar-free goodies, prepare yourself: The Sugar Smart Express Plan allows neither sugar substitutes nor products that contain them. Not even stevia, derived from an herb, which is as natural as it gets. Believe me, I didn't make this decision lightly. In fact, I discussed the merits and drawbacks of allowing sugar substitutes on the food plan with both the nutritionists who developed it and some *Prevention* advisory board members. Lest you think I'm a meanie, let me explain why fake sweeteners didn't make the cut. There are actually two good reasons.

They bait-and-switch your taste buds. Sugar substitutes deliver hundreds of times the sweetness of white table sugar, with few or no calories. Evidence suggests that exposing your taste buds to these high-intensity sweeteners makes them less receptive to natural sources of sweetness such as fruit. For example, sucralose (marketed as Splenda) is 600 times sweeter than sucrose; stevia, 200 to 300 times as sweet. Neotame, a relatively new zero-calorie sweetener, is more than 7,000 times sweeter than white table sugar! High-intensity sweeteners undermine sugar freedom because they reduce your appreciation for the true taste of sweet—the kind that comes from actual food rather than from vats in industrial parks.

They've been linked to an increased risk of obesity and type 2 diabetes. The theory is that exposing our bodies to sweetness without calories can lead to an outpouring of insulin, thereby leading to insulin resistance. For example, a study published in *Diabetes Care* found that diet soda drinkers had an increased risk for type 2 diabetes, and several large studies have associated the use of artificial sweeteners with weight gain.

Even if you're a fan of diet drinks, artificially sweetened yogurt, or those pretty pastel-hued packets that you stir into your coffee, you likely won't miss them for long. According to our test panelists, once their taste buds were "rebooted," the flavor of whole foods and natural sweeteners seemed incredibly intense. "I had an orange with my lunch—it was as sweet as candy!" one of our panelists, Robyn, said. If some of these self-described "sugar addicts" were able to dial down their sweet buds, so can you!

SUGAR MIMICS: WHITE FLOUR AND "FAUX GRAINS"

Foods such as crackers, pretzels, chips, bagels, white rice, and pasta don't always taste sweet and may not even contain sugar. But all are refined carbohydrates, which are digested just as quickly as sugar. In fact, when you eat these Sugar Mimics, glucose floods the bloodstream, triggering a rise in the fat storage hormone insulin and disruptions in other hormones that control appetite. Thus, Sugar Mimics have the same negative effects on health as Straight-Up and Secret Sugars. And we eat a lot of them.

Since the 1970s, the average daily calorie intake in the United States has risen nearly 25 percent. Grains and sugar account for more than half of that increase. We eat 11 servings of grains and grain products on average per day—about twice as many as we should, according to the government's dietary guidelines. Most of those servings come in the form of refined grains, meaning that the grains were processed extensively between harvest and landing in your shopping cart. This category includes "the whites"—white flour, white rice, and pasta and bread made with white flour.

Shockingly, the refined-carbs category also includes what I call *faux grains*—processed whole grain products such as whole wheat bread as well as whole grain crackers, tortillas, and cereals including instant oatmeal, whole grain flakes, and cream of wheat. You're probably aware that research links a steady diet of refined carbohydrates with overweight and chronic disease. But unless you're a sugar smart shopper, the "whole wheat" bread and "whole grain" products you're putting in your cart may not be much better.

The FDA has a strict definition of whole grains: cereal grains that consist of the intact, ground, cracked, or flaked kernel, which includes the bran (where most of the fiber is), the germ (chock-full of protein and healthy fats), and the endosperm (the starchy innermost portion). (In contrast, refined grains contain only the endosperm.)

Whole grains themselves—brown rice, steel-cut and rolled oats, wheat berries–meet that criterion, and they brim with fiber and nutrients. It takes longer for digestive enzymes in the stomach to reach the starch inside whole grains or grains cracked into large pieces, which slows down the conversion of starch to sugar.

For products such as bread or pasta to be labeled whole grain, the FDA says, the grain can be ground, cracked, or flaked, but it must retain the same proportions of bran, germ, and endosperm as the intact grain. So far so good.

However, in the process of making whole wheat or whole grain flour, the kernels are pulverized practically to dust, so they're digested about as quickly as white flour, table sugar, or HFCS. This means that they can spike blood sugar and insulin levels, leading to hunger and prompting you to reach for more of these foods. You're caught in an unending cycle of cravings and consumption.

On the Sugar Smart Express Plan, you break that cycle. And your smaller belly will prove it. Once you begin to introduce sugars back into your diet, you'll add them slowly and in a particular way, so you can determine how you feel without all of that sugar in your system. I'm pretty sure you'll feel awesome. Your cravings will be history. You'll have traded in those sugar rushes and crashes for the steady energy provided by clean eating and nonfood rewards. And, of course, your jeans will fit the way they used to.

Although you're probably eager to lose weight, it's important not to gloss over what research has revealed about the effects of a high-sugar diet on health. I've alluded to the sugar belly. Now I'll clue you in to the sugar heart, liver, and brain. While modest amounts of sugar can soothe body and soul (a square of good chocolate on a bad day can never be wrong), there *can* be too much of a good thing.

3

Sugar-Belly Syndrome: How Added Sugars Harm Health

Here's a little gem that strikes at the heart of our nation's ongoing sugar overdose. In 1822, it took the average American 5 days to consume the amount of sugar in one 12-ounce can of soda. That quantity of soda typically packs 10 to 12 teaspoons of sugar. Do the math, and back then, the typical American swallowed a bit more than 2 teaspoons of sugar a day.

Today, it's 22 teaspoons a day. That's a 1,100 percent increase. Mind blown.

As I mentioned earlier, evidence is building that a sugar-drenched diet increases the risk of not just obesity and type 2 diabetes, which researchers had long suspected, but also of Alzheimer's, liver, and cardiovascular disease. Indeed, as I write this, a major study led by the federal Centers for Disease Control and Prevention (CDC) concluded that a diet high in added sugars may significantly raise the risk of dying from cardiovascular disease.

The American Heart Association (AHA) sounded the alarm about added sweeteners in 2009, when it issued a scientific statement on their effect on health, with a focus on cardiovascular disease (CVD) and its risk factors. The news was a bitter pill. The added sugars in processed foods–primarily sucrose and HFCS–are likely responsible for our increased calorie consumption and contribute to the twin epidemics of obesity and type 2 diabetes, the AHA said. The statement also issued guidelines for added sugar: no more than 6 teaspoons (100 calories, 25 grams) a day for women, and no more than 9 daily teaspoons (150 calories, 37.5 grams) for men.

Yikes. At 22 teaspoons a day, the average American consumes about three times the amount of added sugars recommended for good health. We need an intervention. Now. Because the majority of those 22 teaspoons–352 calories' worth–ends up on our bellies. And if you imagine all the chronic diseases of civilization–obesity, type 2 diabetes, heart disease, and others–as a target, belly fat would be the bull's-eye.

ANATOMY OF A SUGAR BELLY

Wrapping around the heart, liver, and other vital organs like a boa constrictor, deep belly fat is the connection between a sugar-soaked diet, obesity, and disease. Researchers call it visceral fat. I call it *vicious* fat because it can lead to systemwide mayhem.

Subcutaneous fat is the fat we fret about–the kind that widens our hips, thighs, and butt and causes those annoying bra rolls. Located just beneath the skin, subcutaneous fat provides padding and insulation and is a storage depot for energy.

Visceral fat is a different story. This deep belly fat is what researchers call metabolically active, meaning that it churns out nasty substances that impair the healthy functioning of the liver, pancreas, heart, brain, and even women's breast tissue.

For example, deep abdominal fat secretes inflammatory proteins called cytokines. The ongoing slow burn of chronic inflammation has emerged as a link between obesity and insulin resistance, diabetes, and cardiovascular disease.

Science hasn't found such risks in those with curvy hips and thighs. In fact, large studies involving both men and women show that people who store most of their fat in these areas tend not to get obesity-related diseases such as diabetes and heart disease. And a study published in the *International Journal of Obesity* found that gluteofemoral fat—an elegant term that simply means butt and thigh fat—actually traps the fatty acids produced by belly fat and prevents them from doing their damage.

For women, that protection wanes after menopause, as their estrogen levels fall. Their naturally pear-shaped, estrogen-plumped bodies take on more of an apple shape, as fat accumulates around their middles.

How does belly fat develop? It begins with your body's ability to balance glucose and insulin. During digestion, your body breaks down food into its individual components: namely amino acids (from protein), fatty acids (from fat), and glucose (from carbs). Your muscles and brain rely on glucose for energy. Insulin is a hormone that is released by the pancreas to help move glucose from the bloodstream into the cells that use it. The more glucose in your blood, the more insulin you require.

There's where problems can start. Carbohydrates that are digested quickly flood the blood with glucose and result in a large output of insulin. Which carbs are digested quickly? I'm sure you guessed that sugar is one of them. But so are refined carbs. For instance, the kind of whole wheat bread typically used for sandwiches and white bread are digested at about the same rate and cause about the same rise in blood glucose levels, and therefore require the same amount of insulin to clear the bloodstream of glucose.

Over time, continual spikes in insulin have several detrimental effects. First, your cells become less responsive to it. This condition, called insulin resistance, results in your pancreas producing even more insulin to compensate. Glucose levels remain high, and in large amounts glucose can damage blood vessels and nerves.

On top of that–and here's the link to your sugar belly–all that extra insulin floating around causes your body to store more fat than it normally would. It also prevents your body from using fat for energy between meals. Metaphorically speaking, that insulin puts fat in lockdown–once it enters, it's not coming out. And because your body isn't able to use stored fat for fuel, you get hungrier, more often. You produce more insulin, you store more fat. The more fat you have, the more your cells become resistant to insulin. It's a vicious cycle.

Insulin resistance promotes fat storage everywhere. Fructose, on the other hand, contributes to belly fat specifically, according to some studies. It's found naturally in fruits and some veggies that are packed with vitamins, minerals, phytochemicals, and fiber. As any nutrition expert would tell you, though, fruit salad isn't the problem.

The real issue: The amounts of fructose we're consuming in added sugars, such as table sugar (cane or white sugar) and HFCS, are swelling our bellies and menacing our health.

Our bodies were designed to handle fructose in small amounts (for instance, in a few servings of fruit or a little honey a day), not the 60 pounds of high-fructose corn syrup a year the average American consumes, often unknowingly. And in this form, you aren't getting any of the good stuff along with it.

Too much fructose takes a toll on even the youngest hearts, according to a study published in the *Journal of Nutrition*. The study found that teens who consumed the most fructose had higher blood pressure and blood sugar levels than those who ate the least, and it linked high-fructose diets to increases in visceral fat.

Health in America: Sickly Sweet

I'm imagining the added sugars in our food supply—white sugar, powdered sugar, cane crystals—as a gentle snowfall. As the flakes blow in the wind, I stick out my tongue to catch a few. Sweet! But those feathery flakes keep falling, faster and faster. Suddenly, I'm in a bona fide blizzard.

This is the state we all live in today. A blizzard of sugar in our food, threatening to bury us. A flood of HFCS in our beverages (and foods), threatening to take us under. In the past 30 years, as our sugar consumption skyrocketed, so did rates of obesity and other chronic diseases. Evidence is building that this isn't a coincidence. Consider the statistics.

Overweight/Obesity

In 1980, obesity rates—which had held steady in the 20 years prior—rose significantly. Until 1980, just 15 percent of American adults had a BMI above the 85th percentile, suggesting either overweight or obesity. Now, it's 55 percent.

Type 2 Diabetes

In 2010, the annual number of new cases of diagnosed type 2 diabetes was almost triple the number of new cases in 1990.

Heart Disease

While death from cardiovascular disease fell nearly 33 percent from 1999 to 2009, it still accounted for nearly one in three deaths. And projected increases in obesity and type 2 diabetes, among other factors, may slow that positive change in heart health to only 6 percent.

Metabolic Syndrome

In 1990, an estimated 50 million US adults had metabolic syndrome. In 2000, that figure rose to 64 million, a 28 percent jump. A 2010 study revised that figure upward yet again—to 68 million, a further increase of 6 percent.

SUGAR-COATED LIVER DAMAGE

The supermarket is an awesome place to school your kids on healthy eating. But it can get heated if you happen to be in the cookie aisle.

Recently, my son and I were rolling our cart past those sugary squares and disks and double-stuffed whatevers when he informed me that his friend gets *seven* cookies in his lunch every day. (My kids get two, max. After dishes and homework.)

I saw my opening. "Well, let me tell you about nonalcoholic fatty liver disease," I said. Too soon for a 12-year-old? Heck no! I'll tell you what I told him: Overdo the cookies or other sugary foods, and your liver takes the fructose hit.

Located on the right side of your abdomen, tucked behind your lower ribs, your liver has a critical job: to turn toxins–both those formed naturally in the body and those that are man-made, such as from medications, street drugs, and alcohol–into harmless substances. The liver uses about 20 percent of the calories you consume to fuel itself and its work, which includes converting proteins and sugars from food into energy for your body, aided by insulin.

A steady diet of fructose-laden foods can cause globules of fat to begin to form in the cells of the liver. Before 1980, doctors rarely saw this fatty buildup, known as nonalcoholic fatty liver disease (NAFLD). Now, it affects 30 percent of US adults. It's worth noting that the rise in the incidence of NAFLD parallels the increase in obesity and diabetes, and that the condition affects between 70 and 90 percent of those who are obese or have type 2 diabetes. In fact, experts consider NAFLD to be a hallmark of metabolic syndrome, a condition characterized by a cluster of obesity-related conditions. (More on that in a bit.)

This buildup of fat in the liver isn't necessarily obvious on your thighs. A 2012 study in the *American Journal of Clinical Nutrition* found that people who ate 1,000 extra calories of sugary foods for 3 weeks saw just a 2 percent increase in body weight, but a 27 percent increase in liver fat.

When you lose weight, liver fat returns to normal levels. But if NAFLD isn't caught in time, the liver can become inflamed, which can lead to a more severe liver condition known as nonalcoholic steatohepatitis (*steato* means fat, and *hepatitis* is liver inflammation). If the inflammation becomes severe enough, scar tissue replaces healthy tissue, impairing the liver's ability to perform its many crucial functions. When that happens, it's called cirrhosis. (Cirrhosis only happens with really severe alcoholism, right? At least that's what I always thought. Now, it appears, an excessively sugary diet could play a role, too. Amazing.) A fat-riddled liver may become resistant to the action of insulin. As the pancreas churns out more and more of this fat-storage hormone to prod the liver into doing its job, insulin levels increase–and so does body fat.

FRUCTOSE: THE FAST LANE TO BODY FAT?

Along with converting the sugars in food into fuel for the body, the liver also turns excess energy into body fat–a process called lipogenesis. There's some preliminary evidence that the body may turn fructose into body fat more efficiently compared to sucrose and glucose.

In a 2005 study that examined the associations between fructose consumption and body fat, German researchers allowed mice to freely drink either plain water or fructose sweetened water for 10 weeks. Though the fructose-sipping mice regularly ate fewer calories from solid food, they gained weight and ended up with 27 percent more body fat than the mice that drank water. Because fructose doesn't need insulin to enter the cells, it floods the body and is quickly stored as fat, the study found.

In another study, on people, researchers at the University of Texas Southwestern Medical Center in Dallas fed "breakfast" to six volunteers. That meal was 8 ounces of lemonade prepared with three different combinations of sugar: 100 percent glucose, an equal mix of glucose and fructose, or 25 percent glucose and 75 percent fructose.

Immediately after "breakfast," the team measured the conversion of the sugars to fat in the volunteers' livers. Four hours later, the study participants ate lunch, which consisted of turkey sandwiches, salty snacks, and cookies. Each volunteer's lunch contained different amounts of sugars

(continued on page 34)

Robyn Endress

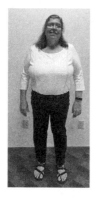

Empowered! That's how Robyn felt after discovering *The Sugar Smart Diet* last year. She had lost 15 pounds on the original 32-day program. Six months later, she was down 61 pounds. "Sugar is my addiction," says Robyn. "When I don't eat sugar, I'm in control. There is a wonderful sense of contentment that pervades my entire body. I can feel hungry, but I don't think I'm going to die if I don't eat something right now. I have absolutely no cravings. I feel satisfied and full after a meal. Food tastes better."

But a few pretzels here, a sandwich on bread there, and the occasional pasta dish and things started to unravel. "I was amazed at how quickly my cravings returned." Robyn regained about 11 pounds, but that wasn't the worst of it. "I felt lousy," she explained. "I had neuropathy back in my feet. My stomach was bothering me. I wasn't sleeping as well." She attributes the problems more to eating refined carbs than to the weight gain.

When the new Sugar Smart Express Plan was announced, Robyn jumped at the opportunity to try it even though she knew it would be tougher because this test panel was during the school year. As a first-grade teacher and single mom of two daughters, Robyn had to juggle all the meal prep with the start of the school year and her daughters' extracurricular activities.

Instead of making a lot of the recipes as she did the first time, Robyn relied on the "create-your-own-meal" formula. On weekends, she'd cook a variety of grains, proteins, and veggies for later use. "Every day, I'd throw a grain like quinoa and a protein like chicken together with some chopped veggies, top it with oil, vinegar, mustard, garlic, salt, and pepper, and voilà—dinner," explains Robyn. "One day, I managed to throw my meal together within 2 minutes before I ran out the door. Two weeks earlier, I would have gone to some fast-food restaurant drive-thru and tried to make the best possible choice."

The effort was worth it. "Within 2 or 3 days of eating no sugar, I found that all the lousy feelings ceased. I felt comfortable in my body once again." The next time she starts to slip, Robyn has vowed "to listen to the signs my body is sending me" and get back on track right away. "My body and my cravings are so much better balanced when I limit the sugars in my diet."

11.7
POUNDS LOST

AGE:
53

ALL-OVER INCHES LOST:
13.5

SUGAR SMART WISDOM:
"Walk, walk, walk! It helps to curb cravings, boosts your energy, and enhances the results of the diet."

Wiped Out by the Fructose Wave

Imagine wading in the ocean, and out of nowhere a huge wave smashes into you, knocking you off your feet. Figuratively speaking, that's how a large influx of fructose hits your liver.

Research suggests that calories from different types of food are metabolized differently in the body. While every one of your body's 10 trillion cells can break down glucose, only the liver can metabolize fructose. Sucrose, or table sugar, is half fructose, so it puts some burden on the liver; the glucose it contains is processed by the rest of the body. HFCS contains about 10 percent more fructose than sucrose, making the liver's job that much harder.

Worse, fructose and other sugars are found in foods that sound healthy. Let's say your standard breakfast is a 16-ounce strawberry-banana smoothie, which you pick up every morning at the local drive-thru. Strawberries. Banana. Only 250 calories. Whole fruit. Sounds healthy. Sweet.

Um, no. That wholesome-sounding smoothie packs 54 grams of sugar, almost all of it added, and the yogurt base contains straight-up fructose. There are other sugars involved, too, and they're not from whole fruit. Don't even get me started on the "strawberry banana fruit base" and "clarified demineralized pineapple juice concentrate."

Your liver must work much harder to break down all that fructose than if you ate a 250-calorie bowl of high-fiber, low- or no-sugar cereal topped with sliced berries. That's because these whole foods contain much less total sugar, and the fiber in the cereal slows the absorption of sugar into the bloodstream. Since the smoothie's sugars come in liquid form, they reach your liver fast.

based on body weight. Then the researchers measured how the food was metabolized.

The results: Lipogenesis rose 17 percent when the volunteers had the fructose-containing drinks, compared to 8 percent for the glucose drink. Simply put, their bodies made fat more efficiently. Further, after metabolizing fructose in the morning, the liver increased the storage of fats eaten at lunch.

As the study's lead researcher, Elizabeth Parks, PhD, put it: "The carbohydrates came into the body as sugars; the liver took the molecules apart like Tinkertoys and put them back together to build fats. All this happened within 4 hours after the fructose drink. As a result, when the next meal was eaten, the lunch fat was more likely to be stored than burned." Although this research is preliminary, it raises important questions about starting your day with a fructose-filled sugary coffee drink or a supposedly healthy fruit smoothie.

According to Dr. Parks, the results of the study likely underestimated the effect of fructose because the volunteers consumed the sugar drinks while fasting, and because they were healthy and lean and could presumably process the fructose quickly. So the fat-packing potential of fructose may be worse if you're overweight because this process may be already revved up.

MAKING THE METABOLIC CONNECTION

I'm no shoe fanatic, but even I get stoked by a BOGO sale–Buy One, Get One Free. Get more of something without paying for it? What's not to love?

Metabolic syndrome gives you the same freebies, but they're usually not anything you actually want. When you have it, you "buy" the extra pounds and net a bundle of nasty, health-threatening conditions at the same time. Belly fat is one of them. Others include high blood pressure, high fasting blood sugar, low HDL ("good") cholesterol, and high triglycerides (fatty substances in the blood).

You don't have to be overweight to have metabolic syndrome, which raises your risk for heart disease, diabetes, and stroke. Up to 40 percent of normal-weight adults have it. But weight isn't the defining characteristic of metabolic syndrome. Insulin resistance is.

A team of researchers, including Robert Lustig, MD, author of *Fat Chance*, advanced a theory of exactly how metabolic syndrome might occur. The process, described in an article published in *Pediatrics,* is extraordinarily complex. But it begins with the body being forced to store excess fat in the liver, as well as in the tissue around the internal organs. This excess fat makes the liver resist the action of insulin. In response, the pancreas produces more insulin to prod the liver into doing its job. Insulin levels rise even higher and cause even more energy to be stored in subcutaneous fat tissue (like your thighs or butt).

The liver tries to export the excess fat that is damaging it in the form of a specific type of blood fat called triglycerides. But too many triglycerides floating around in your bloodstream can be just as problematic. High levels of triglycerides may raise your risk of coronary artery disease, especially if you're a woman.

There's more to this insidious progression of systemwide havoc. But the bottom line is that high insulin levels affect every part of the body–including your belly. In a study published in the *Journal of Clinical Investigation*, 32 overweight volunteers drank either glucose- or fructose-sweetened drinks three times a day and followed a standard diet. The drinks totaled 25 percent of their daily calories.

At the end of the 10-week study, all of the participants had gained weight. But CT scans showed that the fructose group mostly gained belly fat. They were actually growing sugar bellies! On the other hand, most of the glucose group's fat gain was subcutaneous. Compared to the glucose group, the fructose group also had higher total cholesterol and LDL ("bad") cholesterol, plus greater insulin resistance–consistent with metabolic syndrome.

"VICIOUS FAT" AND DIABETES

If a high-sugar diet appears to promote the storage of dangerous belly fat, it's reasonable to conclude that type 2 diabetes can't be far behind. Indeed, research already links sugar intake to the development of type 2 diabetes, independent of its role in obesity. In other words, it's possible that people develop diabetes because they're overweight or obese. But it

The Sugar/Alzheimer's Connection

Research links a nutrient-poor Western-style way of eating with cognitive impairment—issues with thinking, learning, and memory. And we're not just talking the garden-variety brain fart. Research suggests that a steady diet of sugary, processed foods can mess with insulin in the brain. This may trigger what some experts call type 3 diabetes, aka Alzheimer's disease.

Suzanne de la Monte, MD, a neuropathologist at Brown University in Providence, Rhode Island, whose team coined the term type 3 diabetes, was among the first to uncover the link between insulin resistance in brain cells and a high-fat diet. In a paper published in *Current Alzheimer Research*, Dr. de la Monte reviewed the growing body of evidence suggesting that Alzheimer's is fundamentally a metabolic disease in which the brain's ability to use glucose and produce energy is impaired. The evidence, she writes, suggests that Alzheimer's has "virtually all of the features of diabetes [mellitus], but is largely confined to the brain."

In one study, Dr. de la Monte and her team disrupted the way rats' brains respond to insulin. The rats developed all of the brain damage seen in Alzheimer's disease. For example, areas of the brain associated with memory got clotted with toxic protein fragments called beta-amyloid plaques. The rats were unable to learn their way through a maze. In other experiments where insulin resistance was induced, they developed many of the features of Alzheimer's disease.

People with type 2 diabetes are significantly more likely to suffer from Alzheimer's. While the disease doesn't necessarily cause Alzheimer's, researchers believe that both diseases may share the same root: insulin resistance, which can be caused by eating too much sugary, fatty junk food. When researchers fed healthy men and women a high-saturated-fat diet loaded with refined grains and sugary foods for a month, their insulin levels rose—and the levels of beta-amyloid in their spinal fluid rose significantly, an *Archives of Neurology* study reported. A control group on a low-saturated-fat/healthier-carb diet showed reductions in both. Dr. de la Monte's research is ongoing, but the implications are clearly pointing toward an adverse connection between sugar consumption and Alzheimer's.

The best protection against "sugar brain"? Getting sugar *smart*. The Express Plan replaces brain-draining fat and carbs with the nutrients a healthy noggin needs. Of course, your taste buds need love, too. Once you reset them, you'll find that whole, nutritious foods pack the perfect amount of sweetness. You'll experience that for yourself when you start the plan.

may also be possible that they develop it because they're consuming added sugars to excess.

One recent study found an independent, direct link between sugar in the food supply and risk of developing type 2 diabetes. The findings give weight to the still-controversial hypothesis that it's not obesity driving this now global pandemic, but the rising consumption of sugar worldwide.

In this study, published in *PLOS ONE*, researchers from the Stanford University School of Medicine, the University of California, Berkeley, and the University of California, San Francisco, analyzed a decade's worth of health data from the United Nations, including diabetes rates and sugar availability, across 175 countries. After controlling for factors like obesity, aging, income, and total calories, the link between sugar and diabetes remained significant. For every extra 150 calories from sugar available per person each day, diabetes prevalence rises by 1.1 percent, the study found. (By the way, 150 calories is just a little more than the number of sugar calories in a 12-ounce can of soda.) Conversely, reduced exposure to sugar was linked to a drop in diabetes prevalence.

This relationship was unique among food types. Categories such as protein, fat, and fiber didn't show a significant link to diabetes. Neither did total caloric intake.

While the findings don't prove that sugar causes type 2 diabetes, they do support the ever-expanding body of research–in test tubes, animals, and humans–that suggests sugar affects the liver and pancreas in ways that other types of foods don't. Another study, published in *Global Public Health*, found that as a nation's fructose intake rises, so do levels of type 2 diabetes.

Again, the study didn't prove a direct cause-and-effect link, but it did conclude that the prevalence of type 2 is about 20 percent higher in countries where use of HFCS is high, compared to nations where consumption is lower.

SUGAR GOES TO YOUR HEART, TOO

Heart disease has been the leading cause of death in America for almost 90 years—since flappers discovered the Charleston. However, the CDC study I mentioned at the start of this chapter seems to be the very first to suggest that a steady diet of added sugars may lead to heart disease and, well, you know, kill you.

This was a study of more than 30,000 people, based on data from the National Health and Nutrition Examination Survey (NHANES) from 1988 to 2010. The data tracked such things as diet, body mass index, cholesterol level, and blood pressure, as well as behaviors like smoking, exercise, and alcohol consumption. It found that those who got 17 to 21 percent of calories from added sugar had a 38 percent higher risk of dying from cardiovascular disease compared to those who consumed 8 percent of their calories from added sugar. (To put these findings in perspective, on average, Americans get 16 percent of their total calories from added sugars. So this means that most of us should be worrying about this increased risk!)

Other studies suggest that a high-sugar diet does nasty things to your blood vessels, too. For example, high insulin levels cause the smooth muscle cells around each blood vessel to grow faster than normal. This growth tightens artery walls, promoting high blood pressure and thereby raising the risk of heart attack and stroke.

Added sugars in processed foods may also increase cholesterol. A study in the *Journal of the American Medical Association* analyzed 7 years of data from the NHANES. After excluding people with diabetes and high cholesterol, and those who were excessively overweight, the researchers found that adults consumed an average of 21.4 teaspoons of added sugar a day. Alarmingly, as the number of added-sugar calories increased, the levels of HDL cholesterol went down, and LDL cholesterol and triglyceride levels went up. These associations held true even after the researchers controlled for other risk factors for high cholesterol and heart disease. How and why added sugars increase cholesterol aren't yet clear, but one theory is that they cause your liver to secrete more "bad" LDL cholesterol and interfere with the body's ability to get rid of it.

As worrisome as the effects of a high-sugar diet on health are, there's good news: This does not have to be you. At all. Cravings can be crushed–cold. Whole foods can be satisfying *and* a pleasure to eat. You can enjoy all of sugar's pleasures with none of its downsides. Reset your taste buds, and a whole new world of flavor opens to you.

Right now, it's like your tongue is wearing a fuzzy sweater. On this plan, that sweater comes off, and your taste buds are flooded with the delectable, straight-from-nature flavor and sweetness of whole foods. One of our test panelists, Donna, coined a new word to describe the meals on the plan: "yum-o."

Rest assured, yum-o is in your very near future. Before you begin the plan, there's just one more thing to understand about sugar: why we're so drawn to it.

Sugar on the Brain: Cravings, Crashes, and "Addiction"

Cravings happen. Get chocolate, or ice cream, or pizza on the brain, and you can't rest until the first sugary, fatty, delectable bite hits your tingly taste buds.

Defined as an intense desire for a particular food, a craving can be as torturous as the whine of a mosquito in the dark. People who aren't plagued by them often say that cravings are "all in your head." As we discussed in earlier chapters, feelings *can* trigger cravings for specific foods, often those remembered vividly and fondly from childhood.

But there's evidence that food cravings may have a *biological* basis as well: Research suggests that, along with fat and salt, sugar tweaks the reward circuitry of the brain. And some people say they feel compelled to eat sugar, leading some researchers to question whether sugar can be as addictive as drugs or alcohol.

In other words, sugar cravings may in fact be "all in your head"–specifically, in your brain. They may be the result of how the hardwiring of the brain intersects with your life's experiences with sugar.

YOUR BRAIN'S "PARTY CENTRAL" PATHWAY

There are areas in your brain where the pursuit of pleasure meets the drive to survive. These areas are collectively known as the hedonic pathway, or the brain's reward system. Goose this pathway to pleasure with natural rewards like food and sex–rewards that we humans are hardwired to pursue–and it lights up like the sky on the Fourth of July. Unfortunately, the hedonic pathway has the same response to artificial rewards such as alcohol, nicotine, street drugs, and yes, sugar. To paraphrase the writer Elizabeth Wurtzel, the hedonic pathway knows just three words: more, now, again.

This "party central" pathway is composed of two brain areas: the VTA (ventral tegmental area) and the NA (nucleus accumbens). This pathway to pleasure is attuned to two brain chemicals, opiates and dopamine. It's important to understand that foods or activities we associate with bliss–say, ice cream or sex–aren't inherently blissful. The real cause of the delight is those pleasure chemicals flooding our brains. The more important of these chemicals is dopamine.

Working in tandem, the VTA and the NA release dopamine, resulting in what researchers call a feeling of reward and we call pleasure. That fluttery anticipation you feel just before you bite into a piece of chocolate cake? Thank your dopamine supply for hot-wiring your hedonic pathway.

Eat sugar-laden treats too often, however, and over time the brain adapts to the surges in dopamine by producing less of it or reducing the

Added Sugars Rev Appetite

As you've learned, the first humans homed in on the sweetest (and therefore most calorie-dense) plants they could find. Given that they didn't know when they'd find food again, this was a wise strategy. But those Stone Age sugar smarts don't play in the modern world. Our ancestors had to forage. Today, we simply feast—anytime, anywhere. Foods packed with added sugars are a short drive, an Internet connection, or even a text away. The worst part: These sugars may be stoking our desire for sugary, high-fat, high-calorie fare.

In a study of how the brain responds to food cues and how that response increases hunger and desire for certain foods, researchers at the University of Southern California found that young women who looked at pictures of cupcakes and other tempting edibles experienced cravings, especially if they drank a sugary beverage at the same time.

In this study, using functional magnetic resonance imaging, researchers measured the brain responses of 13 young women as they looked at pictures of both high-calorie and low-calorie foods. The women's brains were scanned twice as they viewed images of cookies, cakes, burgers, and fruits and vegetables. After seeing all of the images, they were asked to rate their hunger as well as their desire for sweet or savory foods.

Halfway through the scans, the women drank 50 grams of glucose, which is similar to drinking a can of sugary soda. In a separate instance, they drank 50 grams of fructose.

The researchers had hypothesized that the reward areas in the women's brains would be activated as they looked at the pictures of the high-calorie foods—and they were right. "What we didn't expect was that consuming the glucose and fructose would increase their hunger and desire for savory foods," said the study's principal investigator, Kathleen Page, MD. And fructose resulted in more intense cravings and hunger among the women than glucose did. "This stimulation of the brain's reward areas may contribute to overeating and obesity and has important public health implications," she said.

Research is pointing to fructose, in particular, as an appetite-gooser. In a study of 20 healthy people published in the *Journal of the American Medical Association*, Yale researchers looked for appetite-related changes in blood-flow in the hypothalamic region of their brains after they ingested either glucose or fructose. The study's findings suggested that glucose may reduce bloodflow in parts of the brain that govern appetite, which may help inhibit the desire to eat. That wasn't so for fructose, according to the findings.

number of dopamine receptors in the reward circuit. With the impact of dopamine reduced, you need more of the substance to achieve the same dopamine high. This effect, called tolerance, occurs with street drugs. And it may occur with sugar, too. Research shows that sugar triggers the release of opioids and dopamine, as addictive drugs do, and more lab studies on rodents suggest evidence of sugar addiction.

For example, rats given daily access to sugar in the form of a sugar solution, only to have it taken away, binge on the sweet liquid when it's returned to them. When sugar is taken away, their teeth chatter, they develop tremors and the shakes, and, when put into mazes, they demonstrate anxiety–all signs of withdrawal.

After 2 weeks of abstinence from sugar–imposed by the researchers–the rats begin to seek and crave it, as demonstrated by repeatedly pressing a lever to self-administer it. As it turns out, these findings have implications for humans.

CARB CRAVERS MAY "ABUSE" SUGAR AND STARCH

Do you describe yourself as "addicted" to a certain food? Maybe it's a particular candy bar or ice cream. Perhaps it's potato chips or pizza. Whatever the food, using the a-word makes some nutrition experts uneasy. After all, they've said time and again that there's no such thing as a bad food. And they're right–providing you don't eat so much of it that it causes unhealthy weight gain or makes you feel terrible about yourself.

But what if you *do* consume sugar to excess and can't stop, even if you sincerely want to? When you try to kick sweets or comfort food, you get irritable and moody. When you give in and eat them, your portion sizes spiral out of control. Is it possible for people to be literally addicted to sugar?

While there's no simple answer, there's some evidence that *some* people may abuse sugar. Take, for example, a study conducted at the University of Illinois at Chicago of 61 overweight women, all self-reported carb cravers. The carbs these women craved weren't in fruit or grains, but in chocolate, gummy bears, chips, pasta, bread, pretzels–foods high in easily digested carbs and/or sugar.

The researchers wanted to know about carb-rich foods' "abuse potential"–a phrase that refers to a drug used for its positive effects, including sedation, euphoria, and mood changes. Drugs with abuse potential can produce psychological or physical dependence and may lead to addiction.

The findings, published in the journal *Psychopharmacology*, are interesting. Given a choice between either a carb-rich or a protein-rich drink, and with no information about what either contained, most of these carb cravers preferred the carb-rich beverage. But here's where it gets really interesting. The responses of the women who consistently preferred the carb-y beverage indicated a key criterion of substance dependence: tolerance.

The study was broken into two 3-day sessions that occurred over 2 weeks. For the first 2 days of each "exposure" session, researchers asked the women to recall and focus on a sad memory as they listened to classical music shown in previous studies to invoke a feeling of melancholy.

Once they'd lowered their moods, the women were given either the carb drink (100 percent carbohydrate, from a variety of refined sugars) or the protein drink (37 percent whey protein, 0 percent fat, and 63 percent carbohydrates from refined sugars and food starch). Each volunteer was given one of the beverages in a red-topped cup on one day and the other beverage in a blue-topped cup on the other day; the same drink appeared in the same cup color across both weeks. The third day of each session was the test session: After again self-inducing a bad, sad, or low mood, the women were asked to choose and drink the beverage that had most lifted their moods. By a significant margin, the women reported better moods when they drank the carbohydrate drink.

Even more noteworthy: In the women who consistently preferred the carb drink, their liking for it grew over time, whereas the drink's ability to lift their negative mood decreased over time. This suggests tolerance–the need for more of a substance to get the same effect, or when the same amount produces less of a "rush" with continued use.

The study's conclusion: Sugary, starchy foods *do* show abuse potential– in those who crave them. In other words, it's possible to develop a dependence on these foods' ability to alter your mood.

SUGAR MESSES WITH HUNGER HORMONES

Maybe you don't feel that you "abuse" sugar or carbs. When you're blue, you hit the walking path, not the ice cream. When stress builds, you turn to friends and family, not food, to make it through. And you definitely, *definitely* eat healthy. Whole wheat toast and peanut butter for breakfast. A roasted-veggie or grilled-chicken wrap with low-fat dressing for lunch. A typical dinner is either a take-out salad from the supermarket or a low-calorie frozen entrée.

But you're always hungry. So. Damn. Hungry. And the jeans ain't getting any looser. What's going on?

The Froot Loop Effect

In the late '60s, quite by accident, a graduate student in upstate New York discovered that the lab rats in his care went nuts for Froot Loops. So powerful was their lust for the sugary cereal that it drove them into the center of their roomy, brightly lit cages to get to the treat. Any researcher who works with rats knows that rats prefer cramped, dark surroundings.

The Froot Loop epiphany was one budding psychologist's bread crumb on a trail that will someday lead to a full understanding of what happens in the brain to trigger the compulsion to use substances that snare the body and the brain, like sugar. When I'm seriously considering gorging on a sweet treat, it helps to imagine myself as a cute little varmint, jonesing for a Froot Loop fix. Imagining myself a zombified rat, I have to wonder if I'm really going to risk that electrified field for a Froot Loop. Seriously? No way. That mental picture always makes me laugh—and often helps me just say no.

The hard truth is that even if you avoid soda and sweets, if you don't read ingredients lists, you're likely to be consuming Secret Sugar daily, and more than is healthy. Those added sugars can add up fast–and give you the appetite of a sumo wrestler.

In Chapter 2, you learned that added sugars may goose the brain's reward regions and increase desire for sugary, fatty, high-calorie foods. Other studies suggest that chronic sugar intake messes with our brain's ability to tell us to stop eating. Basically, eating too much added sugar allows the fructose in white sugar and HFCS to send your hunger hormones–the ones that tell your brain you're full–into a tailspin.

Here's what's supposed to happen: Your stomach produces a hormone called ghrelin. That's your brain's cue to send out the "chow down" signal. As you eat, your stomach begins the process of digestion, breaking down your meal or snack and converting it to glucose, which enters your bloodstream.

In response to that influx of blood sugar, your pancreas releases the hormone insulin. Insulin in turn triggers your fat cells to send out a third hormone, leptin, which decreases your appetite. Basically, rising leptin lets your brain know that you've had enough, thank you very much, and you can put the fork down and step away from the table.

Here's where things can go right or wrong. If your cells are sensitive to the effects of insulin, your body uses glucose properly, ghrelin and leptin stay in balance, and you are unlikely to overeat. But if your cells resist insulin's effects–which is likely if you're carrying extra pounds or have type 2 diabetes–your appetite doesn't diminish and glucose is more likely to be stored as fat.

In addition, research suggests that consuming large amounts of fructose can wreak havoc on these hormones of metabolism. That's because leptin, insulin, and ghrelin do not respond to fructose as they do to glucose, so your body doesn't know when it's had enough to eat. Without those internal controls–and with a steady diet of fructose foods–you're liable to gain weight. The worst part: The fructose in these foods is often hidden, so you may not even know you're consuming it.

FROM BUZZ TO CRASH: SUGAR, MOOD, AND ENERGY

Ads for granola or energy bars can make me crazy. Especially when they feature athletic types who claim that it's *this* particular hunk of white flour and added sugars, with a few nuts and seeds mixed in, that they reach for as they climb mountains or run across the Gobi Desert or attempt some equally spectacular feat.

"Quick energy" is the siren song of food manufacturers to an exhausted, sleep-deprived nation. It's quick, all right. Sugar can raise levels of the mood-boosting neurotransmitter serotonin in much the same way as a nutritious, fiber-packed bowl of steel-cut oatmeal can. But like a fling on a sun-drenched island, that energy doesn't last. The time from sugar rush to sugar crash? Thirty minutes or less. In this way, sugary pick-me-ups are a setup for fatigue, low moods, and more unhealthy eating.

Here's how. Let's say, needing a jolt of energy, you reach for a Straight-Up Sugar (a coffee drink, your favorite black licorice) or a Sugar Mimic (a bag of pretzels, a package of peanut-butter crackers). Their refined carbs are digested quickly and speed into the bloodstream as glucose. This rapid breakdown triggers a flood of insulin to transport that glucose into the cells. Shortly thereafter, blood sugar levels nose-dive, you get hungry, you reach for another pick-me-up, and the cycle continues. Sugar also triggers the release of serotonin—which regulates sleep as well as mood—causing post-sugar drowsiness. You may crave more sweets to regain that sugar high or brighten your mood.

Sugar's link to full-on clinical depression is complex. One theory about depression holds that it's caused by a deficiency of brain serotonin. Antidepressants such as Wellbutrin and Prozac increase this serotonin. So does eating carbohydrates. People with serotonin-deficient brains may well medicate with carbs, especially sugary carbs. But over time, it takes more and more sugar to achieve the same boost in brain serotonin. Sounds like a great way to pack on the pounds, no?

So in the long run, sugar does not stabilize mood. It drains you and leaves you feeling worse rather than better. This was shown in a study published in the *Public Health Journal*. A group of Spanish researchers examined the relationship between the incidence of depression and eating sugary sweets and fast food in 8,964 people. The researchers collected data on other variables that could influence the relationship between eating habits and depression, including age and sex, BMI and physical activity level, and total calorie intake and healthy food consumption.

After following the group for 6 years and adjusting for the variables noted above, the researchers determined that those who ate the most junk food had a 37 percent greater risk of developing depression compared to those who consumed the least.

If you suspect your love of sugar is messing with your mood, job one is to steady your insulin and blood sugar levels. Big spikes and dips can zoom you to the bright mood and energetic buzz of a sugar high, followed soon after by a crash that leaves you moody and tired. The Express Diet can help get those blood sugar levels rock-steady.

The next chapter lays out the Express Rules—seven steps to nailing the plan, losing the weight you want, and living a sugar-smart life, for the rest of your life. I think you'll be pleasantly surprised by just how simple and pleasure-centered these "rules" are. Nothing hard. Nothing forbidden. Their common theme: saying "yes." Followed faithfully, they're the key that opens the door to the sweet life that awaits you.

Maria O'Connell

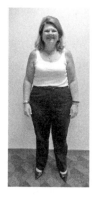

When Maria arrived for her final weigh-in, she strutted in with confidence and excitement. She didn't need a scale to measure her success. The skirt she was wearing said it all. "I could have worn it before if I wanted to squeeze into it, but today it slipped right on," beamed Maria. "I really noticed the inches that I lost in my hips and thighs by the way my clothes were fitting." She lost 2 inches off her waist, 2 off her hips, and 3 off her thighs.

This was a complete 180 for Maria. About 6 weeks earlier, she was frustrated by a lack of results. Since April, she had been walking every day. "I was getting more fit but had not lost any weight," she says.

Things started to click when she shifted her focus to sugar. Up to this point, Maria's attention had been on carbs, which she thought were the culprit for her weight gain. "I was nervous to eat all the quinoa and brown rice because they're high in carbs," she says. "But they taste great, they're filling, and I lost weight."

Cutting out ice cream, granola bars, cereal, cookies, and fruit-flavored yogurt also helped. "Six teaspoons of (added) sugar can be consumed without even tasting it if you are not aware and looking for it," Maria discovered. To get through her 3:00 p.m. witching hour, Maria now sips tea (chocolate-flavored is her new favorite), snacks on almonds, or takes a walk instead of hitting the vending machine.

The good habits are spilling over into other areas of her life, too. Instead of staying up late working, she's going to bed earlier and getting 7 to 8 hours of sleep instead of her usual 4 or 5. "I'm more balanced, I have more energy, and I'm less stressed," Maria says. "Gaining control over my eating has helped me to gain control in other areas of my life. I think more clearly. I work more efficiently. I make better choices." She has even signed up to run her first 5-K.

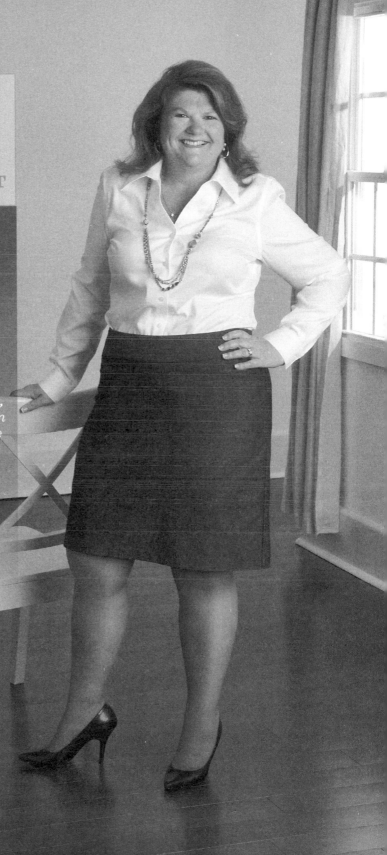

5.6
POUNDS LOST

AGE:
51

**ALL-OVER
INCHES LOST:**
8.25

**SUGAR SMART
WISDOM:**
*"Savor treats like
dark chocolate.
Instead of chewing it,
let it dissolve slowly in
your mouth to get the
full pleasure. Dark
chocolate never
tasted so great—and
you're satisfied with
just a small piece."*

The Sugar Smart Express Rules

Over the next 3 weeks, as you break sugar's grip on your mind and body and shrink your sugar belly for good, these seven rules will keep you on track. They're also meant to encourage positive change not just in your eating habits, but in your life.

A few of these rules address practical stuff, like eating the right foods in the right ways and getting physically active. But most simply point you toward the sweet life. While we all have our own vision of what that is, these rules can help bring it into focus for *you*. They encourage you to savor the little pleasures. Embrace those things that bring you joy, but step out of your comfort zone from time to time to find new delights. Commit to honest to goodness, once and for all, taking care of *you*–your body, yes, but also your heart and soul.

Do sugary treats have a place in the sweet life? Absolutely! The funny thing is, the sweeter your life, the less you tend to crave them. If you have an intense emotional bond with sugar, follow these rules faithfully (especially #4, my personal favorite). They'll help you replace the pleasure or comfort you used to get from sugar with nonfood rewards. Don't be surprised if they start to stir or satisfy cravings in your heart that you didn't even know were there.

This is certainly what happened for me. When I redefined my relationship with sugar, life changed. Cravings-free for the first time, *I* was calling the shots, not sugar. In fact, the less I obsessed about it, the sweeter life got, because thoughts about candy bars and doughnuts weren't taking up space in my head. Today, there's no resentment when I choose not to eat sweets, and no guilt when I choose to splurge. With my daily intention to guide me, I feel like each day, I'm a little closer to achieving a Gandhi-esque harmony in what I think, say, and do. And yes, in what I eat, too.

Our test panelists' success stories reflect this kind of positive change, too. Now it's your turn. Here's a snapshot of you, 21 days from now: Smaller belly. Outsize energy. Less stress. More bliss. And *no more cravings.* You're free. When sugar isn't everything, you can do anything.

EXPRESS RULE #1
Fuel up—and crush cravings—with a high-protein breakfast.

As a working mom, I have plenty of mornings when I don't have time to eat breakfast. But I take the time, because if I skip my morning meal, come midmorning, cravings will come a-calling. Five minutes with a bowl of oatmeal with low-fat milk or a serving of plain yogurt with fruit seems a small price to pay to avoid them.

Besides quelling cravings, breakfast each day keeps the belly at bay. Among people who have lost weight and kept it off, eating breakfast is a common habit. Conversely, people who skip it are 4.5 times more likely to be obese than those who eat it, a study in the *American Journal of Epidemiology* found. Another Harvard Medical School study found that eating breakfast led to better blood sugar control, cutting in half the odds of having high glucose levels.

What you eat is important, though. Start your day with a bowl of cold cereal (even whole grain), a bagel, a muffin, or some fruit, and chances are you will be ravenous in just a few hours. Those meals are primarily carbohydrates—and quickly digested ones at that. Glucose levels spike and insulin is released; soon glucose levels drop precipitously and you're left scrounging for something else to eat.

The antidote: Protein-load your morning meal. Protein slows digestion, and research shows that calorie for calorie, protein is more filling than carbohydrates or fat. Researchers at Saint Louis University found that overweight women naturally took in about 160 fewer calories at lunch when they ate protein-packed eggs in the morning versus a bagel.

Other research shows that protein in the morning makes it difficult for sugar cravings to take hold later on. University of Missouri researchers had 20 overweight young women who routinely skipped breakfast either eat one of two morning meals, cereal or eggs and beef, or no breakfast at all for 7 days. On that last day, the women took part in a 10-hour test that included an all-you-can-eat dinner of microwaveable pizza pockets, as well as an unlimited evening snack of foods such as cookies, cakes, apple slices, and yogurt. The results? The high-protein egg-beef group produced less of the hunger-stimulating hormone ghrelin and more PPY (a hormone that, like leptin, signals fullness) than those who ate cereal. MRI scans showed reduced activity in areas of the brain associated with cravings. In the end, the protein group reported a 30 percent increase in feelings of fullness and consumed 170 fewer calories from their evening snack smorgasbord.

Breakfasts on the Express are hearty—around 300 calories, with at least 20 percent of those calories coming from protein. Your breakfasts will include plenty of lean-protein items, from Greek yogurt and peanut butter to eggs and low-fat cheese. (If you haven't tried the fluffy, high-protein grain called quinoa, you're in for a treat!)

Can't stomach food too early in the morning? No problem. Eat it by 10:00 a.m. and breakfast will still help quell late-day cravings.

EXPRESS RULE #2
Skip work, skip rope, but never skip a meal.

We've all missed a meal because life looks upon our best-laid plans and laughs. Your pet is sick, and it's either lunch or the emergency vet appointment. A commitment that was supposed to take an hour turns into three, your schedule topples like a Jenga tower, and you fall into bed without dinner. Sometimes you just aren't hungry when lunch or dinner or snack time rolls around (rare, but it happens), so you think, no big deal—I'll skip it and save a few calories.

But there's danger in meal skipping—weight and sugar-belly peril. If you cut down on the amount of food you eat for an extended period of time, your body is going to slow things down to conserve its energy supply. If you're looking to flatten your sugar belly, that "starvation response" is the last thing you need. Meal skipping is also a guaranteed way to fire up sugar cravings. Skipping meals lowers blood sugar levels and causes you to overeat the rest of the day to make up for missed calories.

However, we're predicting that you won't want to miss any meals or snacks while you're following the Express Plan. Made with nourishing and delicious whole foods—such as whole grains, beans, lean meats/poultry/fish, nuts, unsweetened low-fat dairy, eggs, and veggies—Express meals and snacks will fill you up and give you the ideal balance of lean protein, energizing carbohydrates, and healthy fats to steady your blood sugar and insulin levels and extinguish cravings for sugar.

EXPRESS RULE #3
Flavor-bomb your taste buds.

As delightful as it is, sugar always tastes basically the same, with variations on *yum, that's sweet*, and *yikes, that's sweet!* But flavor? Ah, an altogether different thing, diverse and surprising. If you've ever dropped a sprig of fresh rosemary into a bottle of extra-virgin olive oil, minced a bundle of cilantro for homemade salsa, or whipped up a from-scratch Indian curry, you know how much flavor fresh herbs and spices add to everyday fare. And as you'll learn, some spices, like vanilla and cinnamon, can put your sweet tooth to sleep, which can help you stick to a healthy eating plan.

The dried herbs and spices in your spice rack are the workhorses of everyday cuisine, but when a dish calls for fresh herbs, do your best to use them. Leafy basil, cilantro, parsley, mint, dill, and thyme are far more flavorful than their dried counterparts. And when you chop them, the fragrance they release is an olfactory delight.

And don't forget other flavor boosters—balsamic vinegar, lemon and orange peel, roasted peppers, hot sauce, toasted nuts, and sugar-free salsa, to name a few. One of my favorites is extra-virgin olive oil. I love its grassy, fruity flavor on salads and vegetables and in soups; even a little drizzle gives me that "I'm full" feeling. I used to think that was because of the fat, but get this—the oil's aromatic compounds seem to be a factor that makes it so satisfying. Just getting a whiff reduced the number of calories people consumed at a meal and even improved their blood sugar response, according to a study from the German Research Center for Food Chemistry. Amazing!

As you move through the phases of the plan, identify which flavors thrill your taste buds and commit to exploring the diverse array of flavors that nature offers. Have you drizzled really good balsamic vinegar over poached pears? Have you grated fresh ginger or chopped citrus-scented cilantro to create a homemade salsa? Enjoy the spiciness of freshly cracked pepper on your salads, or treat yourself to fresh vanilla beans. Stir your coffee or tea with a stick of cinnamon. Toss a serving of plain, air-popped popcorn with a teaspoon of smoked paprika—its deep color and intense flavor go way beyond what you get from the regular type. The more adventuresome you are, the more you'll grow to appreciate flavor and the easier it will be to put sugar in its rightful place in your daily diet.

Sleep Your Way to Sugar Smarts

To many of us, sleep is like an IRS refund check: We never get as much as we need. But there's a good reason to hit the pillow at a decent hour each night: Sleep appears to help sync the hormones that regulate hunger and satiety.

One of the primary goals of the Sugar Smart Express Plan is to restore harmony among insulin, the hormone ghrelin (which triggers appetite), and leptin (which signals satiety). When these hormones are in sync, you tend to experience fewer cravings and are less likely to store fat. But getting less than the recommended 7 to 9 hours of shut-eye may work against you. In research conducted by the University of Chicago, just a few sleepless nights dropped leptin levels by 18 percent and boosted ghrelin levels by about 30 percent. Those two changes shifted appetites into overdrive, and cravings for sugary foods (such as cookies and bread) jumped 45 percent.

Not getting enough shut-eye may not only make sugary, fatty foods more appealing. It may also make it harder to resist them, according to a preliminary study presented at a 2012 annual meeting of sleep researchers.

The parts of your brain that usually put the brakes on cravings aren't as active when you're tired, research conducted at the University of California, Berkeley, found. Scientists had 16 people rate their desire for various foods—once after a night of normal sleep and once after 24 hours without sleep—as they administered brain scans. The volunteers expressed a stronger preference for junk food when they were deprived of sleep. But the scans didn't just show more activity in reward regions. They also showed less activity in regions involved in decision making. The upshot? When you're tired, you may be drawn to sugary, fatty foods partly because your ability to process information and make sound decisions is impaired.

There's nothing more natural than falling into a deep, sound sleep at the end of a brutal day. Yet our tech-heavy, stressful routines conspire to rob us of this simple pleasure. Fortunately, each phase of the Express Plan offers easy ways to de-stress, so you can slip into the restful slumber you deserve—every night.

EXPRESS RULE #4
Live intentionally, every day.

If life is a journey, then today is a day trip, with sights to see and unexpected stops for joy and growth along the way. On the Sugar Smart Express Plan, to make the most of this 24-hour jaunt, you'll set a *daily intention* each morning.

A daily intention is a personal goal for the day that starts with, "Today I will . . . " And they reveal a lot about who you are and what's important to you. A daily intention can be as modest as, "Today, I will walk after work" or as big as, "Today, I will start the process of going back to school." Given shape by daily intentions, your life can become more meaningful and adventurous. You'll start to savor making and following through on them, and sugar becomes just another pleasure, rather than the only one.

It took me a while to learn the importance of setting a daily intention. I figured it out one morning at 5:00 a.m. As was my habit, I was checking my e-mail while waiting for my coffee to brew. (I can get a lot of e-mail overnight!) This particular morning, I had a lightbulb moment: Why was I starting my day with a slew of other people's to-dos at the top of my own to-do list? Then and there, without realizing it, I set my first daily intention: to spend that 5:00 a.m. quiet time on me.

Now, as my coffee brews, I read, meditate, do yoga, or just think about my personal priorities, from big-picture goals to what I need to accomplish that morning. My daily intention can be as practical as, "Today I will order that book on Amazon I've been meaning to read," or as lofty as, "Today I will not let fear motivate me–I will move toward bringing more joy and happiness in my life." This hour of "me" time has made a real difference in my life–every day.

Beginning in Phase 1, you'll set an intention before you begin your day. I'll explain how in Chapter 7, but for now, know this: You'll come to rely on those few minutes, which are completely and entirely all about you and your success.

Nora Haefele

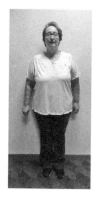

Nora had lost 35 pounds and nearly 18 inches after following the original Sugar Smart Diet for 6 months. "It was a miracle diet for me," says Nora, who has type 2 diabetes and struggled for years to lose weight. While her blood glucose levels were in the healthy range at her 1-year Sugar Smart check-in, she had regained a few pounds. "Not as bad as I thought," she says, but she knew that she was off track. "I wasn't eating cake or cookies or candy," she explains. "I was even very good about avoiding processed snacks like pretzels and crackers. But I would panic if I ran out of pickles! I was stopping on my way home from work because 'I needed pickles.'" An ounce of bread 'n' butter pickles can pack 1½ to 2 teaspoons of sugar.

Nora's backslide started in June during a 7-day kayak trip when she indulged in ice cream, cake, and doughnuts. "It was so easy for so long," Nora says. After the original Sugar Smart Plan, Nora would think of refined carbs as something she was allergic to. "I would never struggle with having to decide whether or not to eat it. But I made a decision in June that wiped out my way of thinking."

Once Nora started the new Sugar Smart Express Plan, though, it all quickly came back to her—just like riding a bike. "I was surprised at how easy it was once I got started again," she says. Within a few days, the cravings were gone, and Nora no longer felt hungry—a feeling she'd been struggling with for several months.

Nora, who walks or runs races from 5-Ks to half-marathons almost every weekend, also posted her speediest half-marathon time of the year—13 minutes faster! After her last one, she was surprised to not have the rungries—an intense hunger and desire to eat after completing a long-distance event.

"I have a new level of vigilance," says Nora. "I don't want creeping behaviors to ooze in and send me back to where I was. I feel so much better, and I perform better when I eat a healthy, whole food diet without lots of sugars and processed carbs."

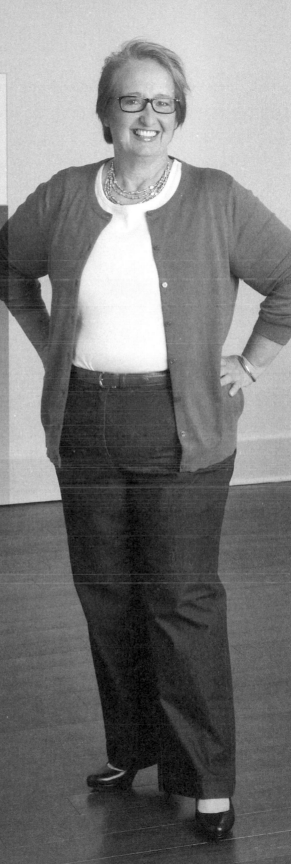

5.8
POUNDS LOST

AGE:
57

ALL-OVER INCHES LOST:
7

SUGAR SMART WISDOM:
"Be meticulous at the beginning of the program. It's hard to reset your taste buds if you cheat even a little."

EXPRESS RULE #5
Inject some joy into each day.

I bet you're thinking, *Perfect! For anyone with the time to sip margaritas on their own private island. I don't have time to hit the ladies' room. Thanks for the tip, but I've got laundry to do.*

Look, I'm busy, too. But over the years I've learned that you don't "make time." *You take it.* To shrink your sugar belly, a daily shot of "me time" is vital to both health and sanity. Those precious 15 or 20 minutes of joy–a romp with your kid through a leaf pile, a page completed in your scrapbook–stand between you and chronic stress, which can send you straight to the cookie jar.

A daily assault of stress hormones from a demanding job or a life in turmoil, chronic stress affects every cell in your body. That wear and tear comes at a price. Numerous emotional and physical disorders have been linked to stress, including depression, anxiety, heart attacks, stroke, hypertension, digestive problems, and even autoimmune diseases like rheumatoid arthritis.

You may also hit the cookies and ice cream pretty hard. When you're stressed, your body releases the hormone cortisol, which signals your brain to seek rewards. Foods loaded with sugar and fat apply the brakes to the stress system by blunting this hormone. When you reach for food in response to stress, you inadvertently create a powerful connection in your brain. The food gets coded in your memory center as a solution to an unpleasant experience or emotion. Face that same problem again, and your brain will likely tell you, "Break out the cupcakes!"

While you can't banish stress from your life completely, you can create an oasis of calm in your daily routine. Managing your stress requires that you find and maintain a balance between the stressful activities that drain you and the relaxing activities that refresh and renew your body and spirit. In each Express phase, you'll discover stress-management techniques you can build into your day. These simple but powerful strategies don't have to disrupt your busy schedule.

For example, if you like oranges, pick up a bottle of orange-scented aromatherapy oil or spray and treat yourself to a hit of "sweet" without the sugar. In a study published in the *Journal of Alternative and Complementary Medicine*, participants who endured a stressful test felt much less anxious when they sniffed orange essential oil 5 minutes before the exam. Best of all, the effects followed them throughout the day. I've used scent as a stress buster for years–it works! I keep a few aromatherapy sprays at home and in my office drawer and choose depending on my mood: lavender for calming, tangerine to brighten my day, peppermint for energizing. Keeping a scented oil or spray at your desk can truly save the day. When you're in crunch time, pause and take a deep whiff. Bam–the modern-day equivalent of stopping to smell the roses. We have a ton more relaxation strategies in store. Small things can deliver such sweet rewards!

EXPRESS RULE #6
Keep it moving.

Ever notice that we do most of our power eating when our butts are in park? In fact, the more you sit, the hungrier you tend to feel. In a study published in *Applied Physiology, Nutrition, and Metabolism*, sedentary people felt 17 percent hungrier than those who moved around during the day, possibly because inactivity spurs secretion of ghrelin.

While exercise isn't mandatory on the Sugar Smart Express Plan, it is encouraged–and you don't need a gym membership or tons of free time to reap its appetite-crushing power. I mentioned walking earlier, and it's a low-tech way to rev the metabolism and quiet the mind. However, it's equally fine to ride your bicycle, do yoga, or dig in your garden, as long as you do it regularly. The more you move, the less hunger and cravings will bedevil you–and the faster your sugar belly will melt away.

Strength training builds calorie-burning muscle, boosts your body's sensitivity to insulin, and strengthens your bones. Another shout-out for the Sugar Smart Express Workout (page 245): It will help you hang on to the muscle you already have, blow off stress, and give you quick energy that lasts.

Walk Away from Cravings

At times, it's just not a good idea to get between me and a square of my favorite dark chocolate. But the next time a chocolate craving hits, I know exactly what I'm going to do: try to walk it off. As it turns out, a short walk may help short-circuit chocolate cravings, a study published in the journal *Appetite* found.

To observe the effect of physical activity on chocolate cravings, researchers recruited 25 "regular chocolate consumers" for their study. This designation was precise. To get chosen for the study, they had to report scarfing at least 3.5 ounces of the sweet stuff every day. To ignite their volunteers' cravings, researchers had them abstain from their favorite sweet for 3 days and told them not to exercise or have caffeine 2 hours before their test periods.

The research team set up two test sessions and held them on separate days. At the first session, one group of chocolate lovers sat quietly while the other group walked briskly on a treadmill for 15 minutes. At the second session, the walkers sat and the sitters hit the treadmill. During each test session, volunteers filled out a scientific questionnaire designed to assess food cravings but adapted to measure chocolate cravings specifically.

After each session, both groups sat quietly for 10 minutes. Then every volunteer performed two 3-minute tasks, with 10 minutes between each task. In the first, the volunteers took a computerized test known to cause psychological stress. The second task? Testers presented the volunteers with a selection of chocolate bars and asked them to open and handle—but not eat—the bar they'd chosen. (If that's not stressful, we don't know what is!)

Compared to how they were at the start of the study, the walkers' cravings dropped by 12 percent, while the sitters' cravings actually intensified. Like chocolate, exercise may increase the levels of feel-good chemicals in the brain's reward regions, thus reducing a desire for sweets, the study authors said.

Makes perfect sense. More often than not, we opt for a chocolate gorge in a bid to feel better, when we know we'll be consumed by post-chocolate regret later. Skip the guilt and walk straight to the reward: feeling awesome.

EXPRESS RULE #7
Feel before you eat.

We all know that there's a connection between how we feel and what we eat, and that the link between sweets and comfort is powerful. But that link can become more like a ball and chain, especially if you learned to associate food with emotions early in life.

In grade school, did a good report card mean an automatic trip to the ice-cream parlor? That could be why you continue to "reward" yourself with dessert. Did your mom dry your tears with a cookie or three, or do you credit chocolate with helping you survive adolescence? It's possible that you associate sweets with comfort even today. Were sugary treats an important part of a time in your life when you felt safe and loved? Today, they may represent an attempt to return to that oasis of peace and security.

The examples above may hit home or spur you to ask other questions. What does my favorite sweet treat mean to me? What promises does it make? Does it deliver on its promises—or snatch them away seconds after my last bite?

The first step to breaking that emotional connection to sugar is to become aware of the feelings that drive you to it. Not after the fact, but at the very moment you reach for sugar. To get a split second of clarity as your fingers close in on your coworker's candy dish: Why am I reaching for this?

Years ago, in college, I took part in a cognitive behavioral stress-eating study. All the participants were asked to keep a food journal and to write down the feeling that accompanied every decision to eat. I followed those instructions to the letter.

Keeping that diary showed me that I ate a lot of doughnuts—something I already knew. But why? On paper, the reason fairly leaped off the page: Each and every time I'd eaten my favorite doughnut, I'd been stressing about exams.

Later in the study, the leaders taught us a slogan: "Stop. Slow down. Think." I did that, too, and learned to recognize the rush of stress that made my brain switch gears from fretting about exams to plotting a doughnut run to the local Italian bakery, which specialized in extra-thick frosting–the kind so sweet it makes your teeth hurt and your eyes bug out. More important, I learned to respond to my desire for sugar with a question: "Do I really want this, or am I just feeding my stress?"

That phrase, from decades ago, is still embedded in my brain. So today, when I reach for something sweet, it's because I've stopped, thought, and consciously chosen to indulge in the pleasure that a sweet treat offers. And then I savor every bite.

Trust me, you can learn to do the same–and our Sugar Smart Express Countdown can help you begin the process of cutting back on sugar and getting the sweet stuff on your radar in an intentional way. Part action, part reflection, the Countdown offers you an invaluable gift: a deep understanding of the role that sugar plays in your history, your life, and your diet. The best part? We're gonna go nice and easy.

Days 1 to 3: The Sugar Smart Express Countdown

At some point in your life, added sugars snared you. Maybe you learned to prefer sweets or junk food early on. Maybe sugar simply snuck its way into your diet without your informed consent. Either way, your history with sugar has shaped your life (and maybe your body as well).

But that's over. You're done being pushed around by your cravings. Sugar freedom begins with this Countdown.

But no cold-turkey tactics. (Do you think I'm a monster?) Over the next 3 days, you'll taper your sugar intake gradually. This gentle, go-slow approach gives your mind and body time to adjust and gives you time to reflect on the role that sugar has played in your diet and your life. Here's a snapshot of each day of the Countdown.

Day 1: Explore your relationship with sugar. Day 1 is more reflection than action. As you continue to eat your regular diet, you'll begin a food log to help reveal your sugar preferences and patterns. You'll also take a quiz designed to reveal the intensity of your emotional attraction to sugar.

Day 2: Sack Straight-Up Sugars—except for your favorite. You'll identify the sources of Straight-Up Sugar in your house and then box them up for friends or the food bank–except for the one that you really, truly, cannot do without, whether it's vanilla creamer in your morning coffee, gummy worms, or that incredibly glorious chocolate-hazelnut spread. This is your *key sugar source,* and it's A-OK to enjoy it during the Countdown.

Day 3: Toss Secret Sugars and Sugar Mimics. You'll identify and eliminate all sources of these sugars and shop for your Phase 1 menu. You'll also complete a quick project that will teach you to replace the sugary "rewards" your brain clamors for with nonfood pleasures. While you'll bid adieu to your key sugar source tonight, you can look forward to a passionate reunion on Day 17.

One more thing. Because our relationship with sugar is shaped by our personal histories, each day of the Countdown features a section called Our Sugars, Ourselves. Each day, you'll answer a Question of the Day that invites you to explore one key facet of your unique sugar profile: the feelings that trigger your desire for sugary foods, your personal habits of sugar consumption, and identifying–and smashing–your "sugar cycle."

Take a deep cleansing breath, and let's get to it!

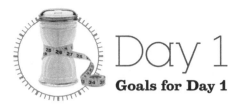

Day 1

Goals for Day 1

- Eat your regular diet and fill out your food log.
- Assess the intensity of your attraction to sugar.

LOGGING YOUR FOOD, LOOKING FOR CLUES

If there's one thing a sugar belly hates, it's emotional awareness in the person it's attached to. To foster this awareness, today and tomorrow, you'll use the food log on page 71 to jot down what you eat for breakfast, lunch, dinner, and every bite and sip in between. I know that keeping a food log isn't everyone's idea of a good time, but please don't skip this step. You won't write pages and pages, you'll keep the log for only 2 days, and you'll learn patterns about your eating habits that will blow you away. One of our test panelists, Joelle, certainly did. To fill out her Day 1 log, she went to the Web site of a national coffee shop to check the nutrition information for her favorite beverage: a chai latte with skim milk. She discovered that the *grande* version she typically orders packs 43 grams of sugar—nearly 11 teaspoons! "That was my eye-opener for the day," she said.

So eat the foods you usually do today. Don't change a thing. That usual morning doughnut or "big grab" bag of chips is *research*! Just note what you eat and the serving size, if possible. Include everything—foods, beverages, sauces, condiments, the spoonful of this and the bite of that. Break out the measuring cups and spoons if you need to. (It's only for 2 days, remember?)

Our food log also has you track your mood and hunger level both before and after you eat. Both will tell you a lot about your emotional and physiological connection to sugar. You'll be able to spot patterns that will raise your awareness of what you eat, when you eat, and why you choose the foods you do. That's the first step to healthy change.

The hunger assessment is simple. Before you eat–meal, snack, or nibble– rank your hunger level on a scale of 1 to 5, and jot down the appropriate number in your log.

1. Starving
2. Hunger pains
3. Hunger
4. Slight hunger
5. Neutral

Then do the same after you eat.

1. Still hungry. You could use a second helping.
2. Full, but not quite satisfied.
3. Content.
4. Stuffed. Your stomach may hurt because it's so full of food.
5. Nauseated. You're so full that you may feel sick.

As I said, there's no need to write a lot. The important thing is to log every bite and briefly recount the circumstances surrounding it. Over the next 2 days, based on these details, a picture of your sugar habits will emerge. Once you're aware of your high-sugar preferences and "sugar cycles"–the times and feelings that prompt you to reach for sugar–you can swap those foods for alternatives that are lower in sugar but still please your "sweet buds" and time your sugar indulgences for maximum pleasure.

For example, you might be shocked to find that although you don't scarf cookies and candy, you're sweet on Sugar Mimics like chips and pizza. Or perhaps you drown most foods in ketchup, which is swimming in Secret Sugars. Every tablespoon of ketchup contains a teaspoon of added sugar. If you're a woman and your log reveals that you typically use 3 table-spoons of ketchup just on scrambled eggs–not hard to do if you don't

(continued on page 75)

Food Log

Please write down everything you eat or drink, including condiments such as ketchup, butter, and sauces. If you eat multiple times between meals, list all items in the same snack row.

For each meal and snack, include serving sizes (measure when possible). From your serving sizes, estimate the grams of sugar you are consuming in these foods. For assistance, look at the item's Nutrition Facts label. Total your grams and divide by 4 to get the number of teaspoons of Straight-Up Sugars you typically eat—there are 4 grams of sugar in 1 teaspoon.

Meal/Snack (please list foods)	Serving Size	Grams of Sugar	Time/ Place	Hunger Level (before/ after)	Moods/ Thoughts
Breakfast:					
After-breakfast snacks, bites, or nibbles:					
Lunch:					
After-lunch snacks, bites, or nibbles:					
Dinner:					
After-dinner snacks, bites, or nibbles:					

Quiz: How Strong Is Sugar's Pull?

Do you and sugar have a bona fide bad romance, or do you simply need to hone your sugar smarts? Take this quiz to find out. Don't feel bad if it turns out that you have a hot-and-heavy emotional attraction to sugar. Once you reset your sugar thermostat, it'll cool down.

   When you finish the quiz, add up your score and compare it to the rankings on page 73.

1. **You find it difficult to say no to your favorite sweets.**
    Always. Place a 4 in column A.
    Usually. Place a 3 in column A.
    Sometimes. Place a 2 in column A.
    Rarely or never. Place a 2 in column B.

2. **If you've tried to cut back on sugar in the past, how intense were your cravings?**
    Very strong. You typically ate what you were craving. Place a 4 in column A.
    Strong, but more often than not, you were able to satisfy your craving with something healthier than what you wanted (for instance, fruit instead of cookies). Place a 3 in column A.
    Noticeable. Sometimes you ate what you were craving and sometimes you didn't. Place a 2 in column A.
    Minor. It took some effort, but more often than not, you distracted yourself and the craving passed. Place a 1 in column B.
    Ignorable. You were able to get past it pretty easily, or you didn't have any cravings. Put a 2 in column B.

3. **You find yourself thinking about sugary foods _____ a day.**
    More than 4 times. Place a 3 in column A.
    3–4 times. Place a 2 in column A.
    2–3 times. Place a 1 in column A.
    Rarely or never. Place a 2 in column B.

4. **Once you start to eat sugary foods, it's hard to stop.**
    Always. Place a 5 in column A.
    Usually. Place a 4 in column A.
    Sometimes. Place a 3 in column A.
    Rarely or never. Place a 2 in column B.

	A	B
1		
2		
3		
4		
5		
6		
7		
8		
9		
10		
11		
	total A	total B
	—	

Add up your score in each column. Subtract your B score from your A score.

5. **Your mood and/or energy level rise right after you eat, but you tend to crash or feel hungry an hour or two later.**

   Always or often. Place a 3 in column A.

   Sometimes. Place a 2 in column A.

   Rarely or never. Place a 2 in column B.

6. **You often feel guilt or shame after you eat sugar.**

   Yes. Place a 2 in column A.

   No. Place a 2 in column B.

7. **You seek refuge in sweets to avoid feelings like anger, loneliness, sadness, or powerlessness.**

   Always or often. Place a 3 in column A.

   Sometimes. Place a 2 in column A.

   Rarely or never. Place a 2 in column B.

8. **You reward yourself with sugar after a challenging task—you feel you "deserve" it.**

   Always or often. Place a 3 in column A.

   Sometimes. Place a 2 in column A.

   Rarely or never. Place a 2 in column B.

9. **You overeat sugary foods when you're under stress.**

   Always or often. Place a 3 in column A.

   Sometimes. Place a 2 in column A.

   Rarely or never. Place a 2 in column B.

10. **At least one of your favorite sweet treats is fused to a memory of feeling loved and cared for.**

    Yes. Place a 1 in column A.

    No. Place a 2 in column B.

11. **The more you indulge in sugar, the less it satisfies—but the more you seem to "need" it.**

    Yes. Place a 2 in column A.

    No. Place a 2 in column B.

Results

A negative number. Your emotional connection to sugar is balanced or nonexistent. But you can still benefit from the Sugar Smart Diet. You may be consuming more sugar than is healthy, either from the Straight-Up Sugars you are eating or from Secret Sugars you may be consuming in amounts far greater than you think. The good news is that you'll have an easy time on the plan.

0–10. You have your occasional struggles with sugar, but overall you have your cravings pretty much under control. You could still be consuming more than you realize, though, and you're likely to notice a difference in the way you feel after following the plan.

11–20. Sugar is one of your go-to coping mechanisms. You use it to soothe or distract yourself, and you're likely consuming much more of it than is healthy. You may have some withdrawal symptoms as you go through the plan, but the strategies I provide throughout will help you take the edge off. You will likely experience noticeable results in your weight, cravings, and mood by the end of Phase 1.

20+. You're very sensitive to sugar's emotional effects and very susceptible to its charms. Phase 1 may be a challenge. But—deep breath—you can reset your sugar thermostat and get back to a place where sugar is a pleasure, not a compulsion. Stick with the plan and you will see dramatic results: The Sugar Smart Diet is your answer to emotional equilibrium and a healthy, happy weight.

Our Sugars, Ourselves

Sweets Emotions

As you've learned, we humans are hardwired to desire sweet foods. So if you swoon for pasta or dessert, relax—you're actually following nature's operating instructions. Because food and socializing/celebrating go together, dining out or special occasions can be especially challenging.

But if a raging sweet tooth leads to weight gain that causes emotional pain, you may be overeating sweet foods not because they're tasty, but because they offer stress relief or emotional comfort.

When the riptide of stress is pulling you under, sugar can seem like a lifesaver. But there's a price to pay: You can begin to associate sweet foods with comfort. Gradually, you may forgo healthier, nonfood ways to relieve stress—a walk, a good cry, a long hot soak—and turn automatically to that sweet shot of instant relief.

Just as sugary foods can temporarily ease stress, they can also soothe uncomfortable feelings you don't want to deal with. People who eat in response to emotions may snack when they're not physically hungry, experience intense cravings for a particular food, and feel unsatisfied even after they finish a hearty meal. They may also eat during or after a stressful experience or to numb their feelings. In a culture that pushes instant gratification, reaching for food is one of the fastest ways to cope with emotions that can be hard to express or even acknowledge.

Question of the Day: Is there a particular feeling that tends to awaken sugar cravings for you? (It might be a negative feeling, like sadness or anger, or a positive feeling, like happiness or contentment.) What is that feeling, and does sugar quell it or amplify it?

_____

_____

_____

_____

_____

_____

monitor portion sizes—you're consuming half of all your recommended daily intake of added sugar in ketchup alone.

Ideally, you'll begin your Day 1 log with breakfast. I suggest making two copies—one for today and one for tomorrow. That way, you can take your log with you and fill it out throughout the day.

If you want to continue the log beyond Day 2, feel free. While you'll follow our tasty menus beginning with Phase 1, you may find that this simple practice keeps you mindful of not only what you eat, but why.

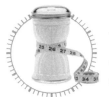

Day 2

Goals for Day 2

- Fill out your Day 2 food log.
- From your Day 1 log, identify the Straight-Up Sugar sources you typically eat.
- Launch Part 1 of the Express Kitchen Cleanup. Eliminate all Straight-Up Sugars in your home except for your key sugar source.

IN THE CROSSHAIRS: STRAIGHT-UP SUGARS

Grab yesterday's food log. Today you're sleuthing out foods that contain Straight-Up Sugar–SUS for short. In your log, write SUS next to each item that you know contains sugar. These foods include:

- Any food or beverage you added white table sugar to–for instance, a few teaspoons in your coffee or tea or on your morning cereal
- Agave syrup, honey, maple syrup
- Sugar-sweetened beverages–soda, juice, lemonade, iced tea, fruit-flavored drinks, chocolate or strawberry milks, sports drinks
- Jams and jellies
- Chocolate and pancake syrups
- Chocolate in its many forms–puddings, snack cakes, candy, cocoa
- Candy–jelly beans, gummy candy, licorice sticks, hard candies
- Sweetened cereals
- Granola or energy bars
- Cookies, doughnuts, packaged snack cakes, frosted toaster pastries, muffins, pies, and other bakery items
- Cake, muffin, or sweet bread mixes
- Ice cream or frozen yogurt
- Yogurt, fruit or flavored

Countdown Cuisine: Sugars Out, Healthy Fare In

On Day 2 of the Countdown, one of our test panelists had tossed out so many of the foods in her house, she didn't know what to eat! Rest assured—I *want* you to eat, and I definitely don't want you to be hungry.

So here's what to eat while you're kicking sugary foods to the curb. Amounts are per meal.

- **Lean protein: 3-4 ounces** skinless chicken breast or thigh; pork tenderloin; shrimp; fish; beef tenderloin, sirloin, or eye of round; or tofu.

- **Veggies: 1-2 cups** broccoli, cauliflower, green beans, zucchini, tomatoes, carrots, mushrooms, onion, asparagus, or eggplant. Salads? Of course.

- **Whole grains: 1 cup** brown rice, wild rice, quinoa, barley, bulgur, farro, teff, or millet.

- **Nuts/seeds: 2 tablespoons** walnuts, cashews, pecans, pistachios, or sunflower, pumpkin, chia, flax, or sesame seeds.

- **Oils/butter: 1-2 teaspoons** olive, canola, sesame, coconut, flax, walnut, or avocado oil or butter.

- **Snack twice a day,** combining a healthy high-fiber carbohydrate (whole wheat bread, cooked whole grains) with protein (turkey or edamame) *or* fat (nuts, nut butters, oils). Stick to ½ cup cooked whole grains, 2 ounces protein, and 2 teaspoons fat/oils.

- **Don't go more than 5 hours between meals.** You want to be hungry for a meal, not ready to gnaw your arm off.

- **Pay attention to how hungry you are before, during, and after your meal** and get adventurous with the Flavor Boosters on page 91. If you're still hungry after a meal, add another serving of veggies and another ounce of lean protein.

- **Sip herbal tea with cinnamon** if you're plagued with sugar cravings at night. The spice helps curb a sweet tooth. Or try a cup of low-fat milk—its protein and fat can help soothe a savage craving.

Count the items that contain SUS and write the number at the top of Day 1. Next, tally the estimated grams of sugar you are getting from these foods, and convert those grams to teaspoons. (Remember that there are 4 grams of sugar in 1 teaspoon.) If you're close to the recommended 6 to 9 teaspoons of added sugar per day, awesome! If not, no worries. Use that number as motivation as you progress through the plan.

Our Sugars, Ourselves

Assessing Our Sugar Patterns

Yesterday, you identified your key sugar source. Today, you'll tease out the details of your desire for it. The when, where, and why, I call them.

Let's say that ice cream is your key sugar source. Your food logs revealed that you enjoyed it at the same time each day: 8:00 p.m. Further, you weren't hungry for it, but your mood was one of contentment and relaxation. In fact, although you've kept your log for only 2 days, you realize that you've followed this pattern for a very long time. But why?

If pressed, you'd concede that you "need" ice cream after dinner. Again, why? After some thought, you may conclude that without that nightly indulgence, you feel deprived. Probe deeper, and you may also realize that it doesn't matter how much sugar you consume during the day, you still want that bowl of ice cream in front of the TV at night.

Knowing the when, where, and why of your desire for ice cream can help you say no to sugary items during the day, for the most part. You realize that these foods don't come close to satisfying you like your nightly dish of ice cream does, and you can make sugar-smart choices based on that knowledge.

Question of the Day: With your key sugar source in mind, determine your unique when, where, and why. Write your answers in the space provided.

- What time of day do you typically eat your key sugar source?

  _____

  _____

- Do you eat it once a day? Multiple times a day?

  _____

  _____

EXPRESS KITCHEN CLEANUP: PART 1

With the exception of your key sugar source, it's time to purge all SUS foods from your refrigerator, freezer, and pantry to make room for the healthy foods in Phase 1 and beyond.

- Do you tend to crave it at the same time each day? If so, what time?

  _____
  _____

- Where do you typically eat it, and what are you doing?

  _____
  _____

- What feeling or mood do you associate with your key sugar source? Tired, overwhelmed, relaxed, content?

  _____
  _____

- Based on your responses above, what circumstances are likely to deliver the *maximum* pleasure from your key sugar source?

  _____
  _____

Did you nail it? Great! If not, worry not. Just return to this question (and perhaps keep your food log) until you have an answer, ideally before you start Phase 4. When you know the when, where, and why of your key sugar source, it's easier to pass up other sugary treats at other times. If you typically have your key sugar source throughout the day, use your answer to help you choose the ideal time to enjoy it once a day.

Tackle your fridge first, followed by your freezer and pantry. Most of the sources will be obvious to you, but refresh your memory if you need to with the list on page 85.

Place all the Straight-Up Sugar sources on your kitchen island or countertops and take one last look. Sure they're yummy. Sure you'll miss them. But these sugary seducers have had their shot–you're moving on! Dispose of them or give them away. But if you wish, keep your key sugar source to enjoy today and tomorrow. (If you'd rather just get rid of it, that's fine, too.)

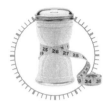

Day 3

Goals for Day 3

- Identify the Secret Sugars and Sugar Mimics you typically eat, using your food logs from Days 1 and 2.
- Launch Part 2 of your Express Kitchen Cleanup. Eliminate all Secret Sugars and Sugar Mimics in your home.
- Make a Rewards Card.
- Shop for Phase 1.
- Toss out your key sugar source by day's end.

TODAY'S TARGET: SECRET SUGARS AND SUGAR MIMICS

Grab your food logs again. Today you're identifying and eliminating foods that contain Secret Sugars and Sugar Mimics. I've combined identifying these two into one step because often the two categories come as a package in foods.

Similar to what you did yesterday for Straight-Up Sugars, place an SS–Secret Sugar–next to all the foods in your logs that you may not think of as containing added sugar, but that do. (On the list below, I've noted which foods tend to contain Secret Sugars, which are Sugar Mimics, and which are sources of both.) Do the same for Sugar Mimics–use SM as your notation. Here's what to look for.

Refrigerator

Ketchup **SS**

Barbecue sauce **SS**

Yogurt, fruit or flavored **SS**

Teriyaki sauce, plum sauce, and other Asian sauces **SS**

Low-fat or fat-free salad dressings and marinades **SS**

Dips and spreads, such as onion dip **SS**

Side dishes from the supermarket deli, such as macaroni salad, potato salad, or coleslaw **SS, SM**

Canned biscuits and pizza dough **SS, SM**

Leftovers from take-out meals, such as pizza or that sweet-and-sour chicken from your favorite Chinese place **SS, SM**

Freezer

Look past the ice cream–if it's still there, it's your key sugar source. Focus on:

Frozen entrées (low-calorie or otherwise) **SS, SM**

Processed meats (sausage, hot dogs) **SS**

Frozen veggies prepared with sauces **SS**

Breakfast sandwiches **SS, SM**

Mini pizza bagels or pizza rolls, or pocket sandwiches **SS, SM**

Frozen bread and rolls **SS, SM**

Potpies **SS, SM**

Pantry

The pantry is a gold mine for Secret Sugars and Sugar Mimics. You'll find them in:

Crackers made with white flour or processed whole grains, such as saltine crackers **SS, SM**

Pretzels, chips, and other salty snack foods **SM**

Pasta sauce **SS**

Pasta, regular and whole wheat **SM**

Couscous **SM**

White rice **SM**

Rice mixes **SS, SM**

Instant flavored oatmeal **SS, SM**

Granola or fruit bars (whole grain varieties included) **SS, SM**

Sweetened cornbread mix **SS**

Whole grain cold cereals (Even the ones that are sugar free and contain fiber are processed and can spike your blood sugar levels. You can reintroduce whole grain cereals with 0 grams of sugar and at least 3 grams of fiber on Phase 2 of the plan.) **SS, SM**

Flour, all-purpose or whole wheat **SM**

Bread, whole grain and white **SS, SM**

Baked beans **SS**

Trail mix **SS**

Whole grain crackers **SS, SM**

English muffins **SS, SM**

Pitas **SS, SM**

Tortilla wraps **SS, SM**

Taco shells **SS, SM**

Rice cakes **SM**

EXPRESS KITCHEN CLEANUP: PART 2

Just as you did yesterday with Straight-Up Sugars, check your logs, count the items that contain SS, and write that number at the top of Days 1 and 2. Do the same for SMs. (If a food is both an SS and an SM, count it only once.) Are you starting to see the type(s) of sugar you typically gravitate to? You're gaining awareness by the day, and that's bad news for your sugar belly.

Now, head to your refrigerator, freezer, and pantry and load up your countertops with the sources of Secret Sugar and Sugar Mimics you find. But this time, there's an extra step. Read the ingredients list on the back of the food's package before you make a decision about what to do with it. Look for sugar by one (or more) of its many names. I listed the various names for sugar in Chapter 2, but I think committing them to memory is so important that I've listed them again in the box on page 85. Not every salad dressing or frozen dinner or what have you will contain sugar. As for Sugar Mimics–those processed grain products, both wheat and whole grain–as I said, most of them (like whole wheat bread, instant oatmeal, and breakfast cereal) contain added sugar as well.

The following foods are reintroduced in Phase 2, so you can stash them in your freezer or pantry if you like until then: tortillas, wraps, pitas, and whole wheat pasta. But as for the others? Dispose of these items in the way you've decided. Toss 'em out, box 'em up, get 'em out–you don't need them anymore. You're taking control of your weight and your health and becoming sugar smart.

Our Sugars, Ourselves

Smashing Our "Sugar Cycles"

Our habits and external cues (TV ads for fast food, smelling cookies you're baking for company) can draw us toward sugar as easily as our food preferences and cravings. These habits and cues can trap us in a vicious "sugar cycle" that we're not aware of.

So can eating sugar out of habit, without really thinking about the why, when, and where. A study published in the journal *Psychological Science* found that people who eat or drink while they're distracted require greater intensities of taste—sweetness included—to feel satisfied. In one part of the study, those who made and tasted lemonade as they memorized a seven-digit number ended up with a 50 percent higher sugar concentration in their drink than when they had to memorize just one number.

Translation? Eating a healthy meal mindfully may make it seem more flavorful. Conversely, paying bills online, watching TV, or fiddling on your tablet as you eat that same meal may make it taste bland and unsatisfying. That's when you may go searching for a sugary hit.

Question of the Day: Look back at your food logs again, think about the triggers that led you to reach for sugar, and complete the worksheet below. You're trying to identify—and smash—any sugar cycles you find. Really try to pinpoint the reason each weak point increases your vulnerability to sugary foods, and come up with solutions. Going forward, you'll find them invaluable when you're in similar circumstances.

Weak Point	When It Occurs	Why It Makes Me "Need" Sugar	Positive Alternatives I Can Use to Meet That Need

Sneaky Sugars Busted! Your "Yep, That's Sugar" Cheat Sheet

Copy this list and take it to the supermarket as you shop for Phase 1 and beyond. Before you buy any processed food, scan its list of ingredients to make sure that it doesn't contain any of the sugars below. Before long, you won't need to take the list—you'll have it all in your head.

Agave nectar
Barley malt
Beet sugar
Brown rice syrup
Brown sugar
Buttered sugar
Cane crystals
Cane juice
Cane sugar
Caramel
Carob syrup
Castor sugar
Coconut sugar
Corn sweetener
Corn syrup
Corn syrup solids
Crystalline fructose
Date sugar
Dextrose
Evaporated cane juice

Fructose
Fruit juice concentrates
Glucose
High-fructose corn syrup
Honey
Invert sugar
Lactose
Maltose
Malt syrup
Molasses
Muscovado sugar
Raw sugar
Rice bran syrup
Rice syrup
Sorghum
Sorghum syrup
Sucrose
Syrup
Turbinado sugar

Linda Kempf

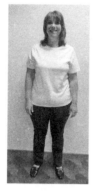

The Sugar Smart Express Plan was a second chance for Linda. About 10 years ago, she had lost 86 pounds, but when she weighed in for the test panel, she was only 10 pounds away from her heaviest weight ever. "With my first weight loss, I didn't change my eating habits," she says. "I exercised a lot, but I wasn't making healthy food choices. I just ate less."

This time, Linda completely revamped how and why she eats. "I had no idea how addicted to sugar I was until I spent 3 days paying attention to what I put into my body," she says. "I thought I was being good by eating the miniature-size Kit Kat bar, but then I'd have four of them. My sugar fix helped me cope when I was stressed or sad. It helped me avoid those feelings."

Besides the obvious sugars in her diet, Linda was surprised to learn how much sugar was in tomato sauce, flavored instant oatmeal, and tonic water. "I was getting 20 grams of sugar in one glass!" Cutting out all of the sugar wasn't as hard as Linda expected because her taste buds quickly recalibrated during Phase 1. "I liked the egg white crepe, but when I made it a few days later, it tasted even better," she explains.

Not only did food taste better and sweeter, but her cravings also disappeared. "After Day 2, I didn't miss my sugar treats!" she exclaims. "It was a shock because I really liked candy. Now I look forward to eating an apple." Plus, she's dealing with the feelings that would drive her to eat by keeping a journal.

The benefits go way beyond the scale. "Even though I'm eating more beans and fiber, I'm less bloated and uncomfortable," she says. "I haven't had to take medication to help me sleep in the past month." And her stamina has skyrocketed. Linda had begun training to walk a half-marathon (13.1 miles) before starting the Sugar Smart Plan. At the time, she was worried about her ability to do it. "I was so tired after a 10-mile walk," she says. But now, "I don't feel as breathless, and my feet and knees don't hurt. When I walked 12 miles last week, I felt good. I think I can do it!"

Linda has the same enthusiasm about maintaining her weight loss this time—and even losing some more pounds! The other day, she noticed the large amount of maple syrup her husband poured on his waffles. "I would have done that in the past, but now I don't need that much to get the flavor. I feel confident that I can make healthy choices and be satisfied."

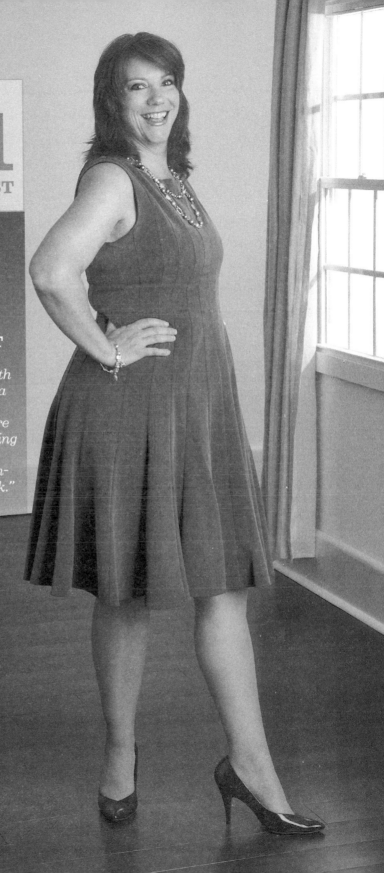

15.1
POUNDS LOST

AGE:
46

ALL-OVER INCHES LOST:
11

SUGAR SMART WISDOM:
"Cook a week's worth of grains like quinoa and bulgur on the weekend. Then store them in single-serving containers for easy use and portion control during the week."

PLEASURE YOUR BRAIN WITH SUGAR-FREE REWARDS

As we now know, highly palatable foods like sweets and refined carbs can activate the brain's reward system, research suggests. To satisfy your pleasure-seeking brain, today you'll create a "rewards card"–a list of nonfood treats that give it (and you) the bliss it seeks, *sans* sugar. From now on, instead of treating yourself to food, you'll treat yourself to a pleasure on your Rewards Card.

Your rewards should be things you can do instantly and that elicit the same pleasure you feel when you indulge in your favorite treat. If you think about it, most of the activities that curl your toes or float your boat are simple and fit into even the craziest schedule. If you're not used to rewarding yourself with anything but sugary treats, consider devoting your daily intention to enjoying one of the pleasures on your card until treating yourself to nonfood pleasures becomes second nature.

Copy the blank form on the opposite page, fill it out, and keep it with you. (Maybe laminate it to make it last.) Whip it out anytime you find yourself craving sugar or refined carbs. Here are some of my personal 20-minute pleasures. Feel free to steal a few for your Rewards Card–but don't pass up the chance to think up your own.

- Watch junky TV
- Watch something silly on YouTube
- Browse a pretty catalog
- Goof off with my kids
- Draw or paint
- Do needlepoint (so relaxing and addictive!)
- Take the dog to the park
- Weed the garden (yes, it's actually relaxing)
- Rake leaves
- Fill the bird feeder and wait for birds
- Give myself a facial

- Finally use those lovely bath salts/scrubs
- Dance like crazy
- Call a really good friend
- Paint my toenails
- Daydream
- Spritz perfume on my wrists or neck
- Take a nap
- Go for a walk, a bike ride, or a run, or stretch
- Pet the cat
- Listen to music
- Plant a flower box for the windowsill
- Plan a dream vacation
- Lie down and look up at the sky

Rewards Card

The pleasure of sugar is fleeting. Instead, I choose to treat myself to . . .

1. _____
2. _____
3. _____
4. _____
5. _____
6. _____
7. _____
8. _____
9. _____
10. _____

When you complete your Rewards Card, practice using it. At some point today (especially if you're stressed), pull out your card, choose a reward, and savor it. Explore the experience throughout the day. How did it feel to take time for yourself? Was your nonfood reward just as pleasurable as, or perhaps even more so than, a sugary treat?

SUPERMARKET ROAD TRIP!

Turn to Phase 1, choose the meals and snacks you want to eat, make out your shopping list, and go! Once you get your groceries home, follow the strategies below to give healthy items prime real estate in your refrigerator, freezer, and pantry, and continue your strategic shelving as you progress through the phases.

Place healthy favorites at eye level. Whether you're opening your refrigerator, freezer, or pantry, your eyes should fall right on the healthy foods you love most. A study that staged a nutritional "intervention" in a large hospital cafeteria, published in the *American Journal of Public Health*, found that making healthy items more visible led people to make healthier choices.

Place veggies, yogurt, and lean protein (such as salmon and grilled chicken breast) front and center in the refrigerator; your air-popped popcorn and rolled or steel-cut oats on an eye-level pantry shelf; and your package of frozen edamame where you'll see it, so you'll remember to thaw it.

Prep now, eat faster later. As soon as you get home from the supermarket, wash, peel, and slice your veggies and place them in see-through containers. Bake your spuds, hard-cook eggs, and prepare grains the night before you plan to eat them. When you walk in the door hungry, you'll be able to whip up a healthy meal without a lot of tedious prep work.

Stash sugars in low places. If your family will continue to eat foods not on your plan, keep their options–especially the sweets and treats–on the bottom shelf of the refrigerator, on the lower shelf in your freezer, and in high or low shelves in your pantry, where you're less likely to see them.

Pantry Check! Common Flavor Boosters to Have on Hand

Chances are, you have many of these in your spice rack, fridge, or pantry already. But it can't hurt to check. We've also included other common items, such as oils, vinegars, and condiments. Today's the day to make sure you have those you plan to use on hand. (You don't have to buy multiple oils and vinegars; it's fine to use those you have.)

Dried Herbs and Spices

- Chili powder
- Cinnamon (or fresh cinnamon sticks, if you have a handheld grater)
- Cumin
- Curry powder
- Dillweed
- Garlic powder
- Ginger
- Nutmeg
- Paprika
- Paprika, smoked
- Pepper, cracked, black
- Pepper, ground, red
- Pumpkin pie spice
- Red-pepper flakes
- Rosemary
- Salt, kosher or plain
- Soy sauce, reduced-sodium
- Tarragon
- Thyme
- Unsweetened cocoa powder
- Vanilla extract (or splurge on whole vanilla beans)

Low-Sugar Flavor Boosters

- Coffee, instant (a small jar will do)
- Enchilada sauce, no sugar added (such as Las Palmas brand)
- Hummus, prepared, any variety (such as Trader Joe's Organic Original Hummus, any flavor of Tribe All Natural, and any flavor of Cedar's All Natural)
- Ketchup (Phases 3 and 4 only—and measure out those portions!)
- Mustard (your favorite— spicy brown, Dijon, etc.)
- Oil, canola
- Oil, olive
- Oil, sesame
- Vinegar, apple cider
- Vinegar, balsamic
- Vinegar, rice

Miscellaneous

- Cooking spray

Shop the European way. Especially if you shop for your family, hit the supermarket more often and buy only for their next few meals, rather than lay in supplies for the week. An overload of choices at home may deplete your willpower, a *Journal of Consumer Psychology* study found.

GET READY TO BLAST OUT OF SUGARVILLE!

Countdown complete–Phase 1 on deck. At this point, you have tossed your key sugar source and stand ready to go stone-cold sugar free for the next 4 days.

Are you fired up? Anxious? Somewhere in between? No matter how you're feeling, I'm with you every step of the way, armed with lots of tools to help prevent and relieve cravings and curb any edginess you might experience. It's also helpful to focus on the benefits you stand to reap 4 measly days from now: looser jeans, renewed energy and positivity, and few to zero cravings for sugar. That's right–you're about to step off the sugar merry-go-round for good.

Just as important, 4 days from now, you'll have altered the way you eat in ways that maybe you thought were impossible. You, passing up your morning bagel or coffee drink or kicking your 2-liter-a-day soda habit? Yes–and that's just for starters. The sweet life is within your grasp. Turn the page and reach for it.

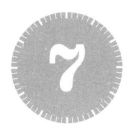

Days 4 to 7: Phase 1

Escape from Sugarville

PHASE 1 GOALS: Reset your taste buds, help your body regain its sensitivity to insulin and maintain steadier blood sugar levels, and set a daily intention each day.

PHASE 1 BENEFITS: By Day 7, you should notice a more positive outlook and energy to burn. You may be sleeping more soundly, too.

Here's the good news about Phase 1: It's short, if not sugary-sweet. And I promise you'll *love* the results. By Day 7, our test panelists lost an average of 4 pounds (one panelist lost 9!) and nearly 4 inches total from their waists, hips, and thighs!

For these 4 days, you will remove all sources of sugar from your diet, even from fruit and veggies such as beets and sweet potatoes. It's the only way to break sugar's grip on you, reset your taste buds, and get your metabolism humming. (Fruit and high-sugar veggies make a comeback in Phase 2.)

During this phase, you'll also remove processed grain products (white and whole wheat) from your diet. This will crush cravings, improve the quality of your diet, and rebalance the way your body uses glucose and insulin. (Hang in there—in Phase 2, bread and pasta are back, in limited amounts.)

For the first day or so, you may feel tired or irritable, and cravings may get intense. Your score on the quiz you took during the Countdown will give you an idea of how strong your sugar cravings are likely to be. On the other hand, you may sail through just fine, as many of our panelists did.

If you *do* experience symptoms, hang tough—they're temporary. It helps to be philosophical, too. As our panelist Nora put it: "If I was allergic to shellfish, I wouldn't struggle with having to decide whether to eat it. I'm approaching sugar the same way."

One thing's for sure—you definitely won't go hungry. Phase 1 meals are designed to keep your belly satisfied, your blood sugar steady, and your cravings at bay. (Some of our panelists couldn't even finish their Phase 1 meals!) Our recipe developers, Stephanie Clarke, RD, and Willow Jarosh, RD, made sure that they contained the right balance of protein, carbohydrates, and fat to prevent the swings in blood sugar and insulin that trigger cravings and promote fat storage.

And as our panelists told us—every day—these meals and snacks are *goood*. Their vibrant, straight-from-nature flavors will dim your palate's demand for sugary fare. You'll find a daily food log with all of your options for Phase 1 on page 98. I encourage you to make four copies of the log and check off what you eat each day.

To manage stress and/or cravings, try the Cravings Crusher tips and Sweet Freedom strategies, which begin on page 116. Use them faithfully, and you create a positive spiral that keeps you on track. And because you'll carry these strategies into later phases, you'll feel more confident and in control with each passing day.

Let's do this!

> For the first time in a while, I am not hungry. —Nora

DO THIS
Phase 1 Strategies

- Set your daily intention each morning (see page 59).

- Have breakfast every morning to help keep cravings at bay. You have four tasty, protein-packed options starting on page 102. Breakfasts have about 300 calories and at least 15 grams of protein.

- Mix and match lunch and dinner options. They're interchangeable from a calorie and a nutritional perspective. Lunches and dinners contain 450 calories and, of course, no added sugar. Have different meals every day, or stick to the three or four you love most—it's up to you. Every meal is easy and quick to prepare.

- We offer two restaurant options in this phase. If you just want a quick and familiar meal, follow the Express "build a meal" formula on page 117, which you can use in any phase.

- Don't forget to snack! Eating every few hours prevents the blood sugar dips that trigger appetite and sugar cravings. You get two snacks a day—one 100-calorie snack and one 150-calorie snack—and you can eat them whenever you want. Just aim to eat something every 4 hours.

- Avoid fruit, fruit juice, dried fruit, sweet potatoes, beets, processed grain products (both white and whole wheat), and, of course, sugar in any of its many forms (including the table sugar you might add to foods, honey, and maple syrup).

- Both avocados and tomatoes—which are technically fruit—are allowed in Phase 1. From a nutritional standpoint, avocados are more like a healthy fat. And both avocados and tomatoes have a much lower sugar content than other fruits, making them more like veggies in that respect.

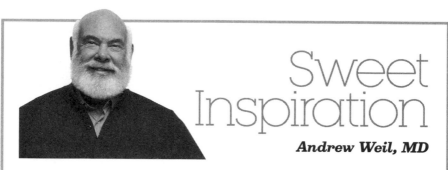

Sweet Inspiration

Andrew Weil, MD

Give your palate an adjustment period. The taste buds soon habituate to a lower overall level of sweetness in the diet—this starts to happen in as little as a week. Foods that once seemed palatable soon seem cloyingly, even sickeningly sweet. A side benefit is that reducing sugar consumption and heightening your sensitivity can reveal a wonderful, subtle sweetness in foods that once seemed to have no sweet notes at all. Certain oolong teas, for example, have a pronounced natural sweetness that I came to appreciate only after I had ratcheted down my consumption of sweet foods.

Eat sugar with a meal, never alone. Generally, the only added sugar I consume is the modest amount that is added to high-quality dark chocolate (70 percent cacao). My reasoning is that the fat in the chocolate slows the spikes and dips in insulin and blood sugar. If you do eat a food with added sugar, the healthiest way to do so is to make sure that the amount of sugar it contains is modest and to have it with foods that are full of fiber, protein, and fat to slow metabolism and control the rise and fall of insulin.

Avoid liquid sugar. The least healthy way to consume added sugar is to drink it in the form of a sweetened beverage. The sugar dissolved in soda is maximally bioavailable. The rise in blood sugar is nearly vertical, and the upcoming dip is correspondingly precipitous.

Eat like it's 1899. Added sugar is a relatively recent invention in human evolutionary history, and we have absolutely no need for it. Added, refined sugar in the diet appeared only in the last 1,500 years or so and in abundance only in the last century. There has not been nearly enough time for human beings to metabolically adapt to consuming copious amounts of sugar. When imagining life without it (or with less of it), imagine yourself as the end product of hundreds of thousands of years of evolution and as a creature exquisitely adapted to thrive on a diet of unprocessed whole foods.

ANDREW WEIL, MD, a leader and pioneer in the field of integrative medicine, is founder and director of the Arizona Center for Integrative Medicine at the University of Arizona in Tucson, where he is also clinical professor of medicine and professor of public health and holds the Jones-Lovell Endowed Chair in Integrative Rheumatology. He is the author of numerous books, including *True Food: Seasonal, Sustainable, Simple, Pure* and *Spontaneous Happiness.*

SHOP THIS
A Shopping List in Each Meal!

The Express Plan allows you to mix and match your meals, so you can customize your shopping list as well as your menu. Here's how.

1. At the start of each phase, choose the meals and snacks you want to eat.

2. Check the ingredients list, which is placed alongside each meal. You'll know right away whether you have the ingredients on hand or need to hit the supermarket. Since you shopped for Flavor Boosters during Countdown, most lists include only main ingredients, such as produce, meats, dairy, and starting in Phase 2 processed whole grain products like breads.

3. Each recipe is a single serving. If you're cooking for two or more, multiply the ingredient quantities by the number of servings you want to make.

As you shop, keep these tips in mind.

- Perpetually pressed for time? Cook grains and chop produce ahead of time.

- You may swap veggies, fruits (in Phase 2 and beyond), whole grains, nut butters, and oils.

- To substitute dried herbs for fresh, use one-third the amount called for. For example, if a meal calls for 1 tablespoon of fresh chopped basil, use 1 teaspoon of the dried variety.

DAILY FOOD LOG

Date:

Today's intention:

Place an X next to the meals and snacks you ate today. You can mix and match your meals and snacks from Phase 1.

BREAKFAST

Hunger level _____

__Basil-Mozzarella Pancakes
__Cinnamon-Vanilla Egg White Crepes
   with Almond Butter Cream

__Mushroom-Sausage Breakfast Bowl
__Pumpkin Spice Oats

LUNCH AND DINNER

Hunger level _____

__Curried Black Bean and Corn
   Burger over Quinoa Salad
__Lemon-Salmon Tabbouleh
__Outback Steakhouse 6-Ounce
   Victoria's Filet, Grilled Asparagus,
   and Baked Potato
__Quinoa Enchiladas
__Southwestern Salad with
   Cilantro Dressing

__Spiced Turkey-Veggie-Quinoa
   Scramble/Wrap
__Starbucks Hearty Veggie and Brown
   Rice Salad Bowl
__Tomato, Onion, and Parmesan
   Salmon Frittata
__Tuna Niçoise Salad
__Turkey Sausage–Mushroom-Onion
   Stuffed Baked Potato with Roasted
   Cauliflower

SNACKS (100 CALORIES)

Hunger level _____

__Asian Edamame and Carrot Salad
__Cumin–Black Bean Dip with Carrots

__Salmon and Corn Salad
__Tomato-Parmesan Bites

SNACKS (150 CALORIES)

Hunger level _____

__Cauliflower Florets and Hummus
__Chili-Spiced Turkey Avocado
   Roll-Ups

__Cinnamon-Walnut Quinoa
__Creamy Kale Salad

DAILY FOOD LOG

ADDITIONAL FOODS

NOTES

FAQs for Phase 1

Q: *These meals contain a lot of sugar. What gives?*

A: As you've learned, grains, beans, dairy products, nuts, vegetables, and milk contain sugar naturally (as do fruits). Not much, mind you, but when you combine foods in a meal, it adds up. Not to worry—none of it is added sugar. Because we created these meals, we know exactly what went into them. We show their sugars per serving to help you get a sense of which foods contain sugar naturally and how much, so you can make healthier choices going forward. Further, knowing the sugar grams in whole foods will help you estimate the added sugars in processed foods. (See page 214.)

Q: *So dairy is okay in Phase 1?*

A: Yes. Milk, cheese, and yogurt contain the natural sugar lactose, which is digested more slowly than other types of sugar and therefore does not have as big an impact on your blood sugar and insulin response. These foods are also packed with protein, which further slows digestion, and calcium, which you need for a healthy heart and bones. And because dairy products don't taste sweet in the way most of us think of as sweet, they're less likely to trigger cravings.

Q: *Why are regular potatoes allowed on Phase 1, and not sweet potatoes?*

A: Unlike a sweet potato, a white potato has very little naturally occurring sugar and doesn't have a sweet flavor that might potentially trigger sugar cravings. Regular potatoes are packed with fiber, which helps moderate the effects their carbohydrates have on blood sugar. Further, some of the starch in potatoes is *resistant starch,* a form of carbohydrate that works in the body much the way fiber does (that is, it is not digested and helps to moderate blood sugar).

Q: *Can I swap ingredients in a meal?*

A: Yes, as long as the ingredients are in the same food group and you're eating phase-appropriate foods. So, for example, you can swap brown rice for quinoa, mozzarella cheese for feta, dairy milk for soy milk, chickpeas for kidney beans, green beans for broccoli, and chicken for fish. Just keep your portion sizes about the same.

Q: *What can I drink in Phase 1?*

A: In all phases, we recommend water, phase-appropriate flavored waters (those in Phase 1 contain no fruit), and unsweetened iced tea or club soda with a slice of lemon or lime. At breakfast, a cup of coffee or tea is fine. Add milk if you like, but no artificial sweetener, sugar, or honey.

Q: *What about alcoholic beverages?*

A: We recommend that you skip the cocktails for the entire 21-day plan. Alcoholic beverages just add extra calories and can make it more challenging to stick with healthy food choices. However, in Phase 2 and beyond you may swap your daily 100-calorie snack for one 12-ounce light beer, one 5-ounce glass of wine, or one shot of vodka, gin, rum, Scotch, or bourbon. Most mixers—even tonic water—have added sugar or are fruit juice–based, so pass on those. Limit your drinks to two per week maximum.

Q: *I have an all-day meeting where lunch will be served, and a wedding coming up. How can I stay on plan?*

A: In any phase, you can build your own meal using the formula on page 117. For weddings or other social occasions, check out our Sugar Smart Express Dining-Out Menu on page 229.

Q: *I blew it! What do I do now?*

A: If you stray from the plan, do not beat yourself up! Get back on track with your very next meal (not the next day). Try to figure out why you got off track, and use those Cravings Crusher and Sweet Freedom strategies!

EAT THIS
Phase 1 Quick & Easy Meals

Have three meals and two snacks every day from the options below.

Breakfast Choices

Basil-Mozzarella Pancakes

Place the oats into a blender and blend until a fine crumb forms, about 30 seconds. Add the egg and milk and blend again until smooth, about 30 seconds. Stir in 2 tablespoons of the mozzarella, 1 tablespoon of the basil, and a pinch each of salt and black pepper. Coat a medium skillet with cooking spray and heat over medium-high heat. Pour in the batter, forming 2 to 3 pancakes, and cook for 6 minutes, turning once. Top the pancakes with the remaining 2 table-spoons mozzarella, the tomatoes, and 1 teaspoon of basil.

Per serving: 287 calories, 19 g protein, 25 g carbohydrates, 4 g fiber, 5 g total sugar, 13 g fat, 5.5 g saturated fat, 413 mg sodium

Shopping list:
⅓ cup rolled oats
1 egg
3 tablespoons fat-free milk
4 tablespoons shredded part-skim mozzarella cheese
1 tablespoon + 1 teaspoon chopped fresh basil
⅓ cup chopped tomatoes

Cinnamon-Vanilla Egg White Crepes with Almond Butter Cream

Whisk the yogurt with the almond butter, almonds, ¼ teaspoon vanilla extract, and ⅛ teaspoon ground cinnamon. Set aside. Whisk the egg whites with ¼ teaspoon ground cinnamon. Spray a medium skillet with cooking spray and heat over medium-high heat. Pour in half the egg mixture. Cook for 3 minutes, or until the crepe turns opaque. Turn and cook for 1 minute, or until cooked through. Repeat with the remaining egg mixture. Fill each crepe with half the yogurt mixture and sprinkle with additional cinnamon.

Per serving: 200 calories, 21 g protein, 13 g carbohydrates, 4 g fiber, 8 g total sugar, 18 g fat, 2 g saturated fat, 223 mg sodium

Shopping list:

⅓ cup low-fat plain yogurt

1 tablespoon almond butter (such as Woodstock Farms, Maranatha, or Artisana)

2 tablespoons sliced almonds

3 egg whites

Mushroom-Sausage Breakfast Bowl

In a medium skillet over medium-high heat, heat 1 teaspoon olive oil. Cook the mushrooms and turkey sausage, stirring frequently, for 5 minutes, or until the sausage is no longer pink and the mushrooms are tender. Remove from the skillet. Cook the egg, sprinkled with a pinch of salt and black pepper, in the same skillet to the desired level of doneness. Place the quinoa in a bowl and top with the sausage mixture. Place the egg on top and garnish with the bell pepper.

Per serving: 298 calories, 19 g protein, 23 g carbohydrates, 3 g fiber, 2 g total sugar, 15 g fat, 3.5 g saturated fat, 486 mg sodium

Shopping list:

⅓ cup sliced cremini mushrooms

1½ ounces crumbled turkey sausage (about ⅓ cup)

1 whole egg

½ cup cooked quinoa

2 tablespoons chopped red bell pepper

Pumpkin Spice Oats

In a small saucepan, whisk the oats, milk, almond butter, and ⅛ teaspoon pumpkin pie spice. Cook over high heat until the mixture comes to a boil. Reduce the heat to medium-low and simmer until the oats are soft and thick, about 10 minutes. Top with the Greek yogurt, a pinch of pumpkin pie spice, and the pecans.

Per serving: 302 calories, 14 g protein, 30 g carbohydrates, 5 g fiber, 10 g total sugar, 15 g fat, 1.5 g saturated fat, 81 mg sodium

Shopping list:
⅓ cup rolled oats
⅔ cup fat-free milk
1 teaspoon almond butter
2 tablespoons 0% plain Greek yogurt
2 tablespoons chopped toasted pecans

"Today, I Intend to . . ."

As I mentioned in Chapter 5, setting an intention each morning helped me put my own health and my well-being first. Today (and every day throughout this plan), set your daily intention. Here's how to do it.

Start with a thank-you. Whether or not you're a person of faith, beginning your day with what you're grateful for sets a positive tone for the entire day. I start my day usually with something as simple as, "Thank you for one more day to be on this planet, seeing my children grow and blossom into the special people that they are."

Select your intention for the day. Once you've given thanks, pick one area of your life that you want to improve or decide on something you want to accomplish. Then create an intention around it. Intentions sound something like this.

Today, I intend to stay aware of how I'm feeling, physically and emotionally.

Today, I intend to do one thing that gives me pleasure.

Today, I intend to start my day with a protein-rich breakfast.

Move into meditation. Just a few minutes of meditation will help you calm your mind and stay focused on the intention you've just set. As you begin your day, you'll feel more centered and less stressed, and you'll have more energy to create a healthy, balanced life you'll love.

Lunch and Dinner Choices

Express on the Go

Outback Steakhouse 6-ounce Victoria's Filet, grilled asparagus, and baked potato (order the Dressed Baked Potato without the toppings and request lemon, salt, and black pepper)

Per serving: 447 calories, 42 g protein, 41 g carbohydrates, 6 g fiber, 4 g total sugar, 0 g added sugar, 9 g fat, 4 g saturated fat, 432 mg sodium

Starbucks Hearty Veggie and Brown Rice Salad Bowl

Per serving: 430 calories, 10 g protein, 50 g carbohydrates, 8 g fiber, 8 g total sugar, 0 g added sugar, 22 g fat, 3 g saturated fat, 040 mg sodium

Curried Black Bean and Corn Burger over Quinoa Salad

In a bowl, mash the black beans. Mix them with the egg, walnuts, ⅛ teaspoon salt, a pinch each of black pepper and garlic powder, and ⅛ teaspoon curry powder. Stir in the corn kernels and form the mixture into a patty. In a small skillet over medium-high heat, heat 1 teaspoon olive oil. Cook the burger for 12 minutes, turning midway. Whisk together 1 teaspoon olive oil, the garlic, 1 teaspoon apple cider vinegar, and ⅛ teaspoon curry powder. Pour the dressing over the cucumber, bell pepper, and quinoa. Serve the burger over the salad.

Per serving: 435 calories, 19 g protein, 45 g carbohydrates, 13 g fiber, 5 g total sugar, 21 g fat, 3.5 g saturated fat, 459 mg sodium

Shopping list:
½ cup black beans
1 egg, whisked
1 tablespoon chopped walnuts
¼ cup corn kernels (fresh or frozen)
¼ teaspoon minced garlic
½ cup chopped cucumber
⅓ cup chopped red bell pepper
⅓ cup cooked quinoa

Lemon-Salmon Tabbouleh

Whisk together 1 tablespoon olive oil, the lemon juice, ⅛ teaspoon salt, and a pinch each of black pepper and ground cumin. Gently toss the bulgur with the salmon, cucumber, tomato, parsley, and the lemon-olive oil dressing.

Per serving: 460 calories, 31 g protein, 40 g carbohydrates, 10 g fiber, 4 g total sugar, 22 g fat, 4 g saturated fat, 771 mg sodium

Shopping list:

2 teaspoons lemon juice

1 cup cooked bulgur

½ cup (1 can) drained boneless, skinless canned wild salmon

½ cup chopped cucumber

½ cup chopped tomato

2 tablespoons chopped fresh parsley

Quinoa Enchiladas

Preheat the oven to 400°F. Mix together the quinoa, onion, bell pepper, 2 teaspoons olive oil, and 2 tablespoons of the mozzarella cheese. Place one-third of the mixture onto the center of each slice of turkey breast and wrap the turkey around the quinoa mixture. Place the 3 wraps in an ovenproof dish. Top with the enchilada sauce and another 2 tablespoons of mozzarella cheese. Bake for 25 minutes, or until steaming hot and the cheese is melted and golden.

Per serving: 454 calories, 33 g protein, 38 g carbohydrates, 6 g fiber, 7 g total sugar, 19 g fat, 5 g saturated fat, 1,240 mg sodium

Shopping list:

¾ cup cooked quinoa

2 tablespoons chopped onion

¼ cup chopped red bell pepper

4 tablespoons shredded part-skim mozzarella cheese

3 slices (1 ounce each) deli turkey breast

¼ cup no-sugar-added red enchilada sauce (such as Las Palmas brand)

Southwestern Salad with Cilantro Dressing

Using a blender or small food processor, blend the cilantro, lemon juice, 2 teaspoons olive oil, a pinch of ground cumin, and ⅛ teaspoon salt for 30 seconds, or until uniform in color and texture. Toss the black beans, corn, and quinoa with the dressing. Serve topped with the tomato and a pinch of black pepper.

Per serving: 440 calories, 17 g protein, 68 g carbohydrates, 16 g fiber, 7 g total sugar, 13 g fat, 2 g saturated fat, 414 mg sodium

Shopping list:

1 tablespoon fresh cilantro

1 tablespoon lemon juice

⅔ cup canned black beans, rinsed and drained

½ cup corn kernels (fresh or frozen)

¾ cup cooked quinoa

¼ cup chopped tomato

Spiced Turkey-Veggie-Quinoa Scramble/Wrap

In a medium skillet over medium-high heat, heat 1 teaspoon olive oil. Cook the bell pepper, onion, and mushrooms, stirring frequently, for 5 minutes, or until the veggies are soft. Add the turkey sausage, ⅛ teaspoon ground cumin, ⅛ teaspoon salt, and ⅛ teaspoon chili powder. Cook for 4 minutes, or until the sausage is cooked through. Remove the skillet from the heat and add the quinoa. Stir gently until heated through. Serve as a scramble or wrap in a collard green, if using, and serve like a burrito.

Per serving: 430 calories, 29 g protein, 40 g carbohydrates, 7 g fiber, 6 g total sugar, 17 g fat, 3 g saturated fat, 986 mg sodium

Shopping list:

½ cup chopped red bell pepper

¼ cup chopped onion

¼ cup sliced cremini mushrooms

4 ounces (about ½ cup) crumbled turkey sausage

¾ cup cooked quinoa

1 collard green, for wrapping (optional)

Tomato, Onion, and Parmesan Salmon Frittata

Preheat the broiler. Whisk together the egg, egg whites, and Parmesan cheese. Stir in the salmon. In a small ovenproof skillet over medium-high heat, heat ½ teaspoon olive oil. Cook the onion for 5 minutes, or until golden brown. Add the tomato. Pour the egg mixture over the onion and tomato and cook for 5 minutes, or until the eggs start to solidify. Place the skillet under the broiler and broil for 3 minutes, or until the egg is firm and golden on top. Serve with the collard greens sautéed in 1 teaspoon olive oil with a pinch of salt, black pepper, and garlic powder and tossed with the bulgur.

Per serving: 470 calories, 50 g protein, 25 g carbohydrates, 7 g fiber, 3 g total sugar, 20 g fat, 5 g saturated fat, 781 mg sodium

Shopping list:

1 egg

2 egg whites

2 tablespoons grated Parmesan cheese

2 ounces (¼ cup) drained boneless, skinless canned wild salmon

2 tablespoons chopped onion

¼ cup chopped tomato

1½ cups chopped collard greens

½ cup cooked bulgur

Tuna Niçoise Salad

Top the spinach with the tuna, olives, grape tomatoes, egg, and potato. Drizzle with 1 teaspoon olive oil mixed with 1 teaspoon apple cider vinegar, ¼ teaspoon mustard (your favorite variety), ⅛ teaspoon dried tarragon, and a pinch of salt.

Per serving: 444 calories, 34 g protein, 32 g carbohydrates, 5 g fiber, 4 g total sugar, 19 g fat, 4 g saturated fat, 773 mg sodium

Shopping list:

1 cup raw spinach

⅓ cup drained and flaked oil-packed tuna

8 halved Greek olives

¼ cup halved grape tomatoes

1 egg, hard-cooked and sliced

1 small yellow potato, baked and sliced

Express Cheat Sheet: How to Cook Grains

Many supermarkets now carry frozen and shelf-stable precooked varieties of brown and wild rice and even quinoa. As long as they're not prepared with any form of sugar, feel free to use them. But if you want to cook whole grains from scratch, this guide can help you cook whole grains like a pro.

Cooking most grains is much like cooking rice. Combine dry grain and water, bring to a boil, and then simmer until the water is absorbed. Sometimes grains aren't tender when their time is up, or are done before the water is absorbed. That's okay. Just add more water and cook until tender, or drain the excess water.

Take note of how much grain you start with (1 cup) and how much you'll end up with. To make less cooked grain, halve the amount you start with and save the extra for the next meal or two. Or cook the full amount to have on hand.

To 1 cup of this grain . . .	Add this much water . . .	Bring to a boil, then simmer . . .	Amount after cooking
Barley	3 cups	45-60 minutes	3½ cups
Brown rice	2½ cups	25-45 minutes (depends on variety)	3-4 cups
Buckwheat	2 cups	20 minutes	4 cups
Bulgur	2 cups	10-12 minutes	3 cups
Farro, whole (not pearled)	2½ cups	25-40 minutes	3 cups
Oats (steel-cut)	4 cups	20 minutes	4 cups
Quinoa	2 cups	12-15 minutes	3-plus cups
Wild rice	3 cups	45-55 minutes	3½ cups

Turkey Sausage–Mushroom-Onion Stuffed Baked Potato with Roasted Cauliflower

Spread the cauliflower onto a baking sheet sprayed with cooking spray. Toss with 1 teaspoon olive oil. Bake at 425°F for 15 minutes, or until golden. With a fork, poke 4 to 5 sets of holes in the potato. Microwave on high until soft, about 8 minutes, turning once halfway through. Slice the potato three-fourths of the way through and gently scoop out half the flesh. In a skillet over medium-high heat, cook the turkey sausage in ½ teaspoon olive oil, stirring frequently, for 3 minutes, or until barely pink. Add the mushrooms and onion and cook, stirring frequently, for 3 minutes. Blend the mushroom mixture with the potato flesh and stuff back into the potato. Serve with the cauliflower, sprinkled with a pinch of salt and chili powder.

Per serving: 457 calories, 29 g protein, 46 g carbohydrates, 6 g fiber, 4 g total sugar, 19 g fat, 3.5 g saturated fat, 875 mg sodium

Shopping list:

1 cup cauliflower florets

1 medium russet potato

4 ounces crumbled turkey sausage

¼ cup sliced cremini mushrooms

1 tablespoon chopped onion

Had to eat dinner at Texas Roadhouse. I went with the filet kebabs, dry baked potato (delish!), and a side of broccoli. Brought half home, so I had a handle on portions, too. I was aware, I had a plan, and I managed it better than I might have in the past. —Donna

---

Fresh Vanilla:
Flavor-Bud Pamperer

Vanilla extract is inexpensive and convenient. That said, if you've never experienced the heady perfume—or taste—of a real vanilla pod, splurging on this scent-sual spice is the perfect way to treat yourself to flavor rather than sugar.

Grown throughout the tropics, vanilla pods, which are the fruit of an orchid vine, look like long, skinny snap beans, with the actual, very tiny beans within. Pollinated and harvested by hand, the pods undergo a lengthy curing process. They're warmed so that they release enzymes that promote flavor and drying, sun-dried to enhance their aroma, and finally dried at room temperature to improve storage.

Suffice it to say, this is a lot of labor. That's why the average two-pack of pods runs around $10 in gourmet shops. But it's this kind of splurge that makes low-sugar eating a true pleasure. Fresh vanilla in my Cinnamon-Vanilla Egg White Crepes or latte? Count me in!

When you get the tough, crinkly pods home, cut them open to extract the beans. Here's how.

Split. With one hand, press the hooked end of the pod to a cutting board to keep it in place. With the other, carefully slice the pod in half with a paring knife, leaving the hooked end uncut. If the pod doesn't split completely, repeat, following your original cut as closely as you can.

Scrape. Continuing to anchor the pod to the cutting board, firmly run the *unsharpened* side of the knife down the pod to remove the tiny seeds, which are more like a paste. Repeat with the other half of the pod. (You use the unsharpened side so that you don't puncture the pod and pull up its fibers.) Most of the beans should be on your knife, rather than on the cutting board or your fingers.

Savor. Most of the meals and snacks that feature vanilla extract call for ¼ teaspoon. The equivalent amount from a vanilla bean: the seed scrapings from a ¼- to ½-inch piece of pod. The more you use, the more intense the flavor.

Save the pod. You can add it to hot tea or warm milk, or to a recipe that requires a heated liquid. Let the pod steep so that it releases all of its delicious flavor.

Store them right. Pods that dry out get brittle and hard to handle, and the beans lose most of their heavenly flavor. Store unused pods in an airtight container, preferably glass, in a cool cupboard.

Snack Choices (1 per Day—100 Calories)

Asian Edamame and Carrot Salad

Whisk 1 teaspoon toasted sesame oil, 1 teaspoon rice vinegar, and a pinch of salt. Toss with the edamame and carrot.

Shopping list:

¼ cup shelled edamame

⅓ cup shredded carrot

Per serving: 103 calories, 5 g protein, 7 g carbohydrates, 3 g fiber, 3 g total sugar, 7 g fat, <1 g saturated fat, 183 mg sodium

Cumin–Black Bean Dip with Carrots

Mash the black beans with ½ teaspoon olive oil, ⅛ teaspoon ground cumin, a pinch of salt, and the lemon juice. Serve with the carrot sticks.

Shopping list:

¼ cup canned black beans, rinsed and drained

1 teaspoon lemon juice

1 medium carrot, cut into sticks

Per serving: 97 calories, 4 g protein, 15 g carbohydrates, 6 g fiber, 3 g total sugar, 2 g fat, <1 g saturated fat, 239 mg sodium

Salmon and Corn Salad

Mix the salmon with the corn kernels, bell pepper, parsley, lemon juice, and a pinch of salt and black pepper.

Shopping list:

¼ cup drained boneless, skinless canned salmon

2 tablespoons corn kernels (fresh or frozen)

1 tablespoon chopped red bell pepper

1 tablespoon chopped fresh parsley

1 teaspoon lemon juice

Per serving: 98 calories, 15 g protein, 5 g carbohydrates, <1 g fiber, 2 g total sugar, 3 g fat, <1 g saturated fat, 375 mg sodium

Tomato-Parmesan Bites

Using a toothpick, skewer a thin slice of Parmesan cheese between 2 cherry tomatoes. Make 2 more mini-skewers, using all the tomatoes and Parmesan.

Shopping list:

3 slices (¾ ounce) Parmesan cheese

6 cherry tomatoes

Per serving: 99 calories, 8 g protein, 4 g carbohydrates, 1 g fiber, 2 g total sugar, 6 g fat, 3.5 g saturated fat, 345 mg sodium

Snack Choices (1 per Day—150 Calories)

Cauliflower Florets and Hummus

Serve the cauliflower florets with the hummus.

Shopping list:

1¼ cups cauliflower florets

¼ cup prepared hummus, any flavor

Per serving: 140 calories, 5 g protein, 19 g carbohydrates, 6 g fiber, 3 g total sugar, 5 g fat, <1 g saturated fat, 186 mg sodium

Chili-Spiced Turkey Avocado Roll-Ups

Cut the avocado into 2 slices. Wrap each slice of avocado with 1 slice of turkey breast and sprinkle with chili powder.

Shopping list:

¼ avocado

2 slices (1 ounce each) deli turkey breast

Per serving: 140 calories, 11 g protein, 7 g carbohydrates, 4 g fiber, 2 g total sugar, 8 g fat, 1 g saturated fat, 578 mg sodium

Had the Cinnamon-Walnut Quinoa snack tonight . . . similar to rice pudding. A fun treat! Very satisfying. —Robin

Cinnamon-Walnut Quinoa

Stir the quinoa and ⅛ teaspoon ground cinnamon into the yogurt. Top with the walnuts.

Per serving: 157 calories, 8 g protein, 17 g carbohydrates, 2 g fiber, 6 g total sugar, 7 g fat, 1.5 g saturated fat, 60 mg sodium

Shopping list:
¼ cup cooked quinoa
⅓ cup low-fat plain yogurt
1 tablespoon chopped walnuts

Creamy Kale Salad

Mix the lemon juice, ½ tablespoon olive oil, a pinch of black pepper, and kale into the cottage cheese.

Per serving: 158 calories, 16 g protein, 7 g carbohydrates, <1 g fiber, 3 g total sugar, 8 g fat, 1.5 g saturated fat, 311 mg sodium

Shopping list:
1 teaspoon lemon juice
½ cup chopped kale
⅓ cup low-fat cottage cheese

My office has this thing called Chocolate Fridays. Today's assortment: doughnut holes, M&Ms, candy, and for the nutrition-minded, bananas. Maybe it's time for one of my snacks. Should I have the Chili-Spiced Turkey Avocado Roll-Ups, or the veggies and hummus? Hmmm ... —Joelle

YOU GOT THIS
Managing Stress and Cravings in Phase 1

Yes, you're eating in a new way. But you still have your old life to contend with—a frantic schedule, constant stress, and constant temptation to give in to your favorite treats. The Cravings Crushers and Sweet Freedom strategies below can help you cope with any cravings that surface and ease the stress that can trigger them.

Cravings Crushers can help you overcome the physical symptoms that may occur when you remove sugar from your diet or better manage your blood sugar levels. Sweet Freedom strategies are so named because they soothe stress or offer emotional comfort better than sugar. (And use that Rewards Card! That's what it's there for.)

If you habitually turn to these tools instead of to sugar, you'll be breaking unhealthy patterns and creating a positive spiral that will motivate you to stay on track. And because you'll carry the strategies you learn each day into the next, your discomfort will ease day by day, replaced by a positive upswing in energy and mood.

Day 4

If you feel a bit nervous today, I understand: Today is D-Day (Ditch Sugar Day). But it's *also* the day you begin to break sugar's grip on your mind and body and kick-start a full-body health revolution.

It's difficult to predict how you'll feel today. At least for today, any desire for sugar will stem more from habit (or resistance) than physiology. While it would be too early for physical symptoms to occur, you may feel strange without your regular go-to sugars within arm's reach. If you get a craving, turn to one of the nonfood rewards on your Rewards Card or today's Sweet Freedom strategy to get the stress relief or emotional comfort you're used to getting from sugary treats.

You might also think about the power of habits today. So many of the food decisions we make aren't decisions at all; we choose certain foods–sugar and refined carbs included–because we always choose them. In this phase, you're learning that consuming sugar is a mindful choice–for pleasure, not out of habit.

Cravings Crusher: Take Out Some Nutrition "Insurance"— A Multivitamin

While supplements can't take the place of a healthy diet, there's some evidence that two nutrients–calcium and vitamin D–may help quell cravings and accelerate weight loss.

Extra body fat holds on to vitamin D so that the body can't use it. This perceived deficiency interferes with the action of leptin, the hormone that tells your brain you're full. In a study of 1,800 overweight people being treated at a weight loss clinic, the heavier the participants, the lower their vitamin D levels tended to be. According to the study, published in the *Journal of Nutrition*, it may be that people who are overweight are less able to convert vitamin D into its hormonally active form.

Moreover, if you're deficient in calcium, your body can experience up to a fivefold increase in the fatty acid synthase, an enzyme that converts calories into fat. In a study published in the *British Journal of Nutrition,* 63 overweight women were put on a 15-week diet and took 1,200 milligrams of calcium and 400 IU of vitamin D a day. The women who had adequate intake of calcium at the start of the study did not see any benefit, but those with low intakes (600 milligrams or fewer)–a situation many women find themselves in–lost six times more weight than women who followed the diet but did not take a supplement.

While you'll get plenty of calcium on this plan, a bit of extra nutrition "insurance" can't hurt. Consider taking a multi that supplies 25 percent of the Daily Value (DV) for calcium (250 milligrams) and at least 400 IU of vitamin D, preferably in the form of D_3 (cholecalciferol), which is better used by the body than other forms. You may find that your cravings fade while your weight loss speeds up.

Plan B: Build Your Own Meal

No time to shop. A business lunch or dinner. Thanksgiving at Aunt Jane's. No worries—you can still follow the Express Plan! Just use the formula below to create your own sugar smart meal. Easy-peasy.

- **4 ounces lean protein (chicken or turkey breast; pork tenderloin, loin, or chops; lean beef like sirloin or eye of round; fish; or tofu)**
- **1–2 cups vegetables**

- **1 cup whole grain** *or* **1 medium potato**
- **1–2 teaspoons butter or oil**
- **2 tablespoons nuts or seeds or ¾ ounce cheese** *or* **3 tablespoons shredded cheese**

Sweet Freedom Strategy: Keep Your Mind on Your Meals

Mindfulness is a way of thinking and focusing rooted in Buddhist meditation. In the West, it's come to mean cultivating a moment-by-moment awareness of your thoughts, feelings, bodily sensations, and environment. When you practice mindfulness, you just accept where you're at in this moment, rather than fret about the past or worry about the future. You can do anything in a mindful way–walk, wash dishes, even eat. Especially eat.

A large body of research has sprung up around mindful eating, and the findings are overwhelmingly positive. Study after study suggests that eating "in the moment" promotes weight loss and healthier choices. When you eat in a mindful manner, you're fully aware of and appreciate the flavors, textures, and aromas of every bite. You're equally tuned in to your thoughts, feelings, and sensations of hunger and fullness. The payoff: You enjoy your food more and don't need as much to feel satisfied.

Starting with your next meal, try mindful eating for yourself. There are many versions of this exercise, but all have a core concept: When you eat, focus on nothing else–no books, phones, or tablets at the table. Always sit to eat, and do nothing but focus on your food, bodily sensations, and thoughts and feelings.

Try this exercise alone a few times, to experience it fully without feeling self-conscious. After a time or two, you should feel comfortable practicing it when you eat with others.

1. Sit at the table, with your plate in front of you. Take several deep breaths to allow your body and mind to settle. *Now* pick up your fork.

2. Look at your food and ponder its origins. The Buddhist monk, teacher, writer, and peace activist Thich Nhat Hanh developed an exercise where you imagine the life cycle of your food. He does a meditation on an orange that I love. You imagine the blossom, envision the fruit growing and ripening, and appreciate how long it took to grow. You contemplate the sun that nourished it, the farmer who picked it, the driver who carried it, the store person who displayed it–all of the phases it has passed through to come to you. You thank them all–the tree, the sun, the people. Gratitude is at the heart of mindfulness.

3. Take a bite, taking time to observe your fork rising to your mouth and your mouth opening to receive it. Notice the shape and size of the morsel, as well as its color, texture, and scent. Place it on your tongue and chew, tuning in to its flavor, temperature, and texture.

4. Chew each bite for at least 20 seconds. By focusing on sensations such as taste and smell, eating–an activity that you may have performed on autopilot for years–can feel brand-new.

5. Notice your thoughts and feelings. Do you like what you're eating? Are you comparing it to previous meals? Do you wish you had more, or are you feeling satisfied?

6. As you finish, take a few deep breaths, then leave the table. Remind yourself of how the plate looked when it was full and how it looks now. When you focus on your food, you're less likely to overeat and consume things that don't truly nourish you.

Sweet Dreams!

Design Your Own Wind-Down Ritual

To give your mind and body time to transition from your active day to bedtime drowsiness, design a personal hour-long bedtime "countdown." My countdown goes like this: An hour before bed, I put away my phone, make a cup of warm milk "sweetened" with a shot of vanilla extract, and watch junky TV with my kids. (Sometimes, I read aloud to them from a low-brow detective novel.) Old ladyish? Perhaps. But so, so soothing.

Not sure how to design your own "countdown"? Try divvying up that hour into two or three 20- or 30-minute increments, and make each relaxing and pleasurable. I've offered a sample bedtime ritual below, but tweak it to fit your own habits and schedule.

9:00-9:20 p.m.: Prep tomorrow's meals. Don't worry about the coming day—keep your head in the moment. Chop fruits and veggies and pack your lunch in a mindful way.

9:20-9:40 p.m.: Do your ablutions. Shower or bathe, brush and floss, moisturize, slip into clean PJs.

9:40-10:00 p.m.: Relax. Do a couple of rounds of circle or yoga breathing (see page 121), then slip between the sheets. No books, phone, or tablet—you want your body to associate bed with sleep only.

Day 5

Have any sugar cravings cropped up? They may not, but it can't hurt to focus today's intention on what you'll do if your taste buds start demanding the sugar-laced favorites they're used to. To quiet those cravings, whip up that protein-packed breakfast, splurge on an item on your Rewards Card, and hang tough. If a craving does hit, it's likely to pass in 15 minutes or less.

Cravings Crusher: Zing Your Taste Buds, Zap Your Blood Sugar

You'll notice that all of our salad dressings in this and subsequent phases are made with fresh herbs, olive oil, and the vinegar of your choice.

Flavorful, yes–but there's another reason to dress those greens with vinegar. In a study published in the journal *Diabetes Care*, people with insulin resistance or type 2 diabetes had lower blood sugar levels when they consumed slightly more than a tablespoon of vinegar immediately before a high-carb meal.

In this study, researchers fed 10 people with type 2 diabetes, 11 people with insulin resistance, and 8 people with no blood sugar issues a sugary, starchy breakfast: orange juice and a bagel, which packed a hefty dose of carbs (87 grams). However, 2 minutes before the meal, half of the participants drank a "vinegar cocktail"–4 teaspoons of apple cider vinegar and a teaspoon of saccharin (which we don't recommend) in an 8-ounce glass of water. The remaining volunteers were given a placebo drink. Everyone's blood sugar was measured both before and after the breakfast.

A week later, the researchers repeated the experiment, with those who'd received the vinegar getting the control drink and vice versa.

All three groups had better blood sugar readings after meals begun with those vinegar cocktails. But those with insulin resistance saw a 34 percent reduction in their postmeal blood sugar levels, while those with type 2 diabetes experienced a 19 percent reduction.

The acetic acid in vinegar may inactivate certain starch-digesting enzymes, slowing carbohydrate digestion, the study's authors said. In fact, the researchers noted that vinegar's effects may be similar to those of the blood sugar–lowering medication acarbose (Precose).

Went to the movies this afternoon. To avoid dipping my hands in my girls' popcorn, I brought both my 100- and 150-calorie snacks. Enjoyed 12 almonds, a light string cheese, and a 100-calorie bag of dry-roasted edamame. I was completely satisfied and didn't feel deprived in the least.
—Robyn

The bright, tart taste of natural vinegar puts the flavor of many of those bottled dressings to shame. You can use any kind of vinegar–red wine, apple cider, or balsamic. Spoon a tablespoon of balsamic over meat or veggies, too, to intensify their natural flavors.

Sweet Freedom Strategy: Circle Breathing

Stress is sweeping over you like a tsunami. Sugar is whispering in your ear. Before you give in, try circle breathing, a simple way to relieve stress fast. When you're anxious, off center, or feeling like you'll explode if you don't have your bag of mini peanut butter cups, do a round of circle breathing 5 to 10 breaths. During Phase 1, aim to use this centering exercise five or more times a day, which will help your body and mind form a strong, positive habit. What's more, according to a recent study in the *Journal of Alternative and Complementary Medicine*, relaxation breathing after meals helps prevent glucose spikes.

1. Inhale and stretch your arms over your head. Exhale, giving a sigh of relief as you lower your arms. Relax and keep your arms lowered for the rest of the exercise.

2. Now imagine that you're inhaling a stream of peaceful energy into a spot a few inches below your navel.

3. Continue inhaling, imagining the energy traveling to the base of your spine. Then imagine it traveling up your back to the top of your head.

4. Exhale, and mentally follow that breath back down the front of your body to the point below your navel where you'll begin the next inhale. Your breath has now made a full circle–up the back of your body, down the front, and back to the starting place below your navel.

5. Do 5 to 10 circle breaths. You can also use circle breaths for a longer period as a relaxing form of meditation.

Day 6

If you're going to experience cravings, they're likely to hit today. You may get a headache, feel more tired than usual, or snap at the people around you. No, it's not fun (for you or for them), but look at it this way: Such symptoms mean that the sugar is leaving your body and will soon make its absence felt in your mood and on the scale, and they aren't likely to last much longer. It's all downhill from here.

Cravings Crusher: Add Some Spice to Your Day

You'll notice that many of our meals include cinnamon and (in later phases) ginger. That's because these warm spices (nutmeg and allspice are others) along with vanilla extract give you tons of flavor with none of the sugar. Plus, they seem to quell a sweet tooth. And cinnamon, in particular, may do even more: In 60 people with type 2 diabetes, just a teaspoon a day for 20 days improved insulin response and lowered blood sugar by up to 20 percent, according to a study published in the journal *Diabetes Care.*

For the best flavor, buy whole cinnamon sticks and grind them in a spice or dedicated coffee grinder. Store the sticks or powder in an airtight container in a cool, dark place. Then try these tasty ideas (if you like things spicy, add nutmeg, too).

- Stir your herbal tea with a cinnamon stick and let it steep as you sip.
- Cinnamon and low-fat dairy were made for each other. In this phase, you're already sprinkling cinnamon over your oatmeal and yogurt. But in later phases, it sweetens up popcorn and part-skim ricotta cheese, which is divine when spread onto whole grain toast. Along with a dash of vanilla extract, cinnamon also sweetens up a pre-bedtime cup of steamed fat-free milk.
- Cook your grains with a cinnamon stick and maybe a bay leaf. It gives them a wonderful depth of flavor.

Sweet Freedom Strategy: Tune In to "Body Hunger" Rather Than "Head Hunger"

Although eating is meant to be a pleasure, it's helpful to know the difference between physical hunger and appetite. I asked you to rate your hunger when you were keeping your food log on Days 1 and 2. It's a good idea to get in the habit of asking yourself "How hungry am I?" before a meal and after–before you reflexively reach for a second helping (or later on, dessert). It may mean the difference between staying on plan or overeating when you're not truly in need of fuel for energy.

Hunger is a physical feeling that develops when you have not eaten for several hours or you skip a meal. Appetite is a psychological feeling, often prompted by the sight or smell of food. For example, you may want a cupcake when you pass a bakery and see them displayed in the window, or you may want dessert even after a large meal.

When you're not sure if you're hungry–which can happen if you're used to eating what you want, when you want it–use the hunger scale in Chapter 6 (on page 70). Taking a few minutes to rate your hunger can help you decide if what you're feeling is true physical hunger or simply a desire to eat for other reasons. It also is helpful to use during a meal to monitor how full you're getting. It's a simple but effective technique.

As you progress through the phases, try to use the scale before and during each meal and snack. Before long, you should be in tune with when you're truly hungry–or when you want to eat because stress, the sight or smell of food, or uncomfortable feelings are pushing your appetite buttons. If you want to lose weight and keep it off, knowing the difference can keep you slim for good.

Day 7

You made it! By this time, most people experience a surge in energy and mood, and the headaches, fatigue, and crankiness have faded away. Continue

Whip Up Some Flavored Waters

You've never tasted water like this—all flavor, and not a grain of sugar added. These tasty libations are sweet stand-ins for the sugary drinks you may be missing right about now. Simply place the ingredients in a 2-quart jar, muddle with a wooden spoon or spatula, cover with 6 cups of ice, fill the jar with water, and stir. Pop it in the refrigerator for 2 hours to chill and let those luscious flavors mingle. Strain, then drink up! Each recipe makes 2 quarts and will keep in the refrigerator for 2 to 3 days. In Chapter 9, I'll introduce more flavored waters, made with sweet and luscious fruit.

Cucumber-Jalapeño Quencher

2 cucumbers, peeled and thinly sliced
2 jalapeño chile peppers, seeded and sliced (wear plastic gloves when handling)

Vanilla Latte

2 vanilla beans
2 cups whole coffee beans

to use the techniques you've learned in this phase as you begin Phase 2 tomorrow. You'll find more tools to help you sail through cravings and really start loving your new, low-sugar life.

Cravings Crusher: Cool Cravings with Water

According to some experts, dehydration can spike cravings for sugar and junk food dramatically—and take a toll on your mood as well. Recent studies have linked mild dehydration to fatigue, anxiety, poor concentration, and even your cranky midday slump.

Despite the frequent bathroom trips, drinking water throughout the day is worth it. It may promote weight loss by speeding up metabolism, according to a study published in the journal *Obesity*. The latest guidelines from the Institute of Medicine recommend that women get 91 ounces of water a day—more than 11 cups! You might be relieved (no pun intended) to know that not all of it has to come from the tap. In fact, at least 20 percent of the water you get will come from food. If you eat lots of fruits and veggies, as you will on this plan, you'll make a hefty dent in your water needs. Coffee and tea count, too. Diet soda, however, does not–and as you've already read, the artificial sweeteners it contains may be a secret plumper-upper. If you're looking for a flavorful libation, try our fabulous flavored waters on the opposite page.

Sweet Freedom Strategy: Strike a Pose to Counter Cravings

Yoga can help relax and quiet your mind, so sugar cravings won't gain traction in your brain. Even the simple physical pose below (called an *asana*) requires you to focus intently on your body and your breathing. This intense body awareness can help calm the mind. Focusing on your breathing can downshift the body's stress response, so you can respond rationally to cravings, rather than react emotionally.

Further, relaxation or meditation can help you begin to tune in to desires that sugary treats can't satisfy–more joy in your life, meaningful work, the courage to follow a dream. Once you're in touch with these desires, you can take steps to make them happen, rather than use sugar to suppress them.

This simple standing forward bend can help you relax and decompress, allowing you to reflect on the emotion that's driving your cravings. Here's how to do it.

1. Stand with your back about a foot from a wall and your feet hip-width apart.
2. Lean back onto the wall. Then gently bend your knees and fold forward, bringing your belly and chest to your thighs. Take 6 to 12 breaths, focusing on the exhalation.
3. Slowly roll up, one vertebra at a time, until your back is leaning up against the wall again. Close your eyes and take a few breaths. Repeat 3 to 5 times.

Alison Ackerman

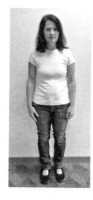

Alison had known that she was a sugar addict for years. When presented with the opportunity to have a cookie or candy, "I would want to say no, but always said yes. It was like I would be missing something if I didn't have it," she explains. "If I fought it and then gave in, there would be that orgasmic rush feeling of the sugar and sweetness hitting my tongue."

Thankfully, running counteracted Alison's sweet tooth—until she turned 40 and went to nursing school. It got worse when she started to work night shifts. "It's hard to not just eat and eat anything and everything when you're up at an unnatural time," she says. Over the next few years, Alison got into a vicious cycle of eating and not exercising and gained about 30 pounds.

This past summer, Alison realized that she needed to slim down to keep up with her four active kids. "The weight was stealing my energy," she remembers. In addition to starting to run again, she also picked up a copy of the original *Sugar Smart Diet*. "I was doing more reading than doing, but I had started to read labels," she says. Those little changes helped her to lose about 15 pounds. Now she was ready to tackle her sugar addiction.

While it was tough at the beginning, especially when she realized that she also needed to cut out refined carbs, the changes she saw kept her going. "Nothing tastes as good as fitting your 43-year-old butt into some skinny jeans," she says. And other benefits were equally motivating. "I haven't gone this long without a headache, ever," says Alison, who used to get two or three headaches a week. Her digestive system also likes her new way of eating. She no longer has to take Prilosec for reflux, and she's less gassy.

Her running has improved, too. "It's easier," she says. "I feel 10 years younger!" And it's noticeable. "People are asking what my secret is!"

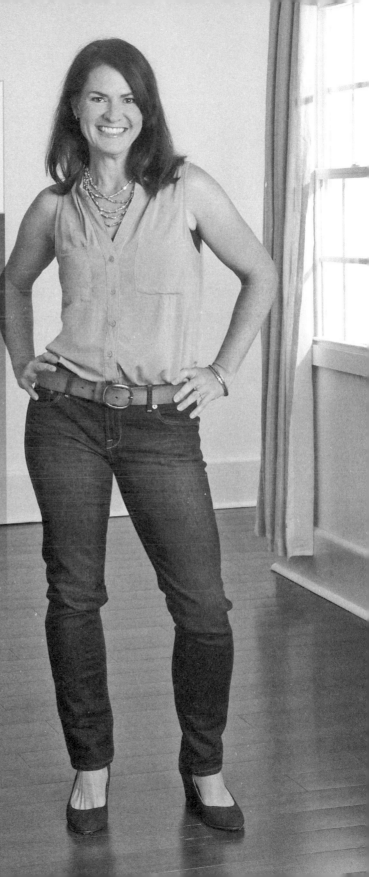

10.7
POUNDS LOST

AGE:
43

ALL-OVER INCHES LOST:
7.75

SUGAR SMART WISDOM:
"Bring your own food. Yogurt, edamame, cheese and grapes, hard-cooked eggs, soup, or other high-protein, high-fiber snacks are good options to have on hand when you know tempting foods will be around."

8

Days 8 to 11: Phase 2
Fruitylicious!

PHASE 2 GOALS: To reintroduce the natural sweetness of fruit to your newly virgin taste buds; intentionally experiment with herbs, spices, and Flavor Boosters; and manage any residual cravings triggered by stress or strong emotions.

PHASE 2 BENEFITS: By the end of this phase, you should have few to zero cravings, combined with more awareness of your unique stress triggers and how to manage them without turning to sugar. If you're walking and/or doing the Express Workout, you may be falling asleep as soon as you hit your pillow, and waking up refreshed.

Eliminating fruit in Phase 1 helped reset your sugar thermostat. By reintroducing it now, while added sugars are still off the menu, you learn what "sweet" really tastes like. When I lived in Poland, where sugary sweets and junk were hard to find, I developed a love for mandarin oranges. Every day, on my way to work, I'd buy a couple of *mandarynki* and sit them on my desk for snack time. There was so much to love–the fact that I could peel them in about 3 seconds, their citrusy scent hitting my nose, their delectable flavor burst of sweet and tart. I'm still crazy about these little fruits–so flavorful and fragrant, so pretty and sugary-sweet.

Think of fruits as crayons. You wouldn't use just red and yellow, right? You want the whole colorful box to pick from. It's the same with fruit. All fruit contains fiber, vitamins, minerals, and various disease-fighting nutrients like antioxidants and phytochemicals. The different colors are indicators of different nutritional profiles. Red watermelon and grapefruit are great sources of lycopene. The dark reds, purples, and purple-blues in fruits like cherries, plums, and blueberries indicate that they're rich in anthocyanins. Mangoes, peaches, nectarines, apricots, and cantaloupe pack carotenoids, such as beta-carotene. The more colors you choose, the more health benefits you'll reap.

What's more, fruit is packed with nutrients and fiber, which slows the breakdown of the food in your digestive system, leading to a far more gradual release of sugar into your body. This means that a flood of glucose does not hit your bloodstream, and your liver is not overwhelmed by fructose. Add to that the fact that studies have directly linked fiber to long-term weight loss. And when you enjoy the sweetness of fruit, you're less likely to reach for processed, nutritionally bereft items. I recently ate a half-cup of fruit salad, which contained in-season blueberries and strawberries, mango, banana, orange, and apple. I kid you not. The sweetness was like fireworks in my mouth. Trust me: Until you've rebooted your taste buds, you cannot imagine the sweetness of fruit.

Feel free to enjoy any Phase 1 meal in Phase 2. That said, we have 20 new meals to tempt your palate–again centered on fresh, whole foods–and three more low-sugar on-the-go meal options. Dig in!

DO THIS
Phase 2 Strategies

- Stick with breakfast. As in Phase 1, start your day with a protein-packed breakfast to keep your appetite and blood sugar on an even keel. In this phase, you'll find some terrific fruit options. When fruit is paired with protein and fat, it's even more satisfying.

- Keep on snackin'. Eat one 100-calorie and one 150-calorie snack at any time. While fruit can be part of your 100-calorie snack, pairing it with protein or fat can make it even more satisfying. See the chart on page 146 for some fruit and protein combos.

- Enjoy three servings of fruit a day. You can have it as a snack, dessert, or as part of a meal. One serving equals a cup of sliced fruit or one medium piece of whole fruit. Stick to those servings–fruit does contain lots of sugar, albeit the naturally occurring kind. If strong sugar cravings have been an issue in the past, you may want to choose low-sugar fruits more often (see the chart on page 146).

- Optional: Enjoy one serving of a processed whole grain product each day. Because it can be difficult to find commercial breads that don't contain added sugar, the options in Phase 2 come in the form of tortillas and pitas, which tend to contain about 1 gram or less of added sugar. If you choose to eat one of our wrap or burrito options, you'll be taking in a minuscule amount of added sugar. If you opt for cereal, pick one with 0 grams of sugar and 3 or more grams of fiber per serving.

- Stay intentional! You may be feeling more in control of your cravings and your diet now, but please continue to set your daily intention. Reminding yourself each morning of your wish to live a low-sugar life, and deciding how you'll do that in a small way each day, can keep you focused and motivated.

- Avoid white flour and products made with it, white rice, fruit juice, and added sugar in any form.

SHOP THIS

Choose your meals and customize your list, just as you did in Phase 1. Each recipe is a single serving. If you're cooking for two or more people, multiply the ingredient quantities by the number of servings you want to make.

DAILY FOOD LOG

PHASE 2

Date:

Today's intention:

Place an X next to the meals and snacks you ate today. You can mix and match your meals and snacks from Phases 1 and 2. Boldface indicates an option added in this phase; an asterisk denotes a recipe that can be found in Chapter 7.

BREAKFAST

Hunger level _____

__Basil-Mozzarella Pancakes*
__**Breakfast Brown Rice Fritter**
__Cinnamon-Vanilla Egg White Crepes with Almond Butter Cream*
__**Creamy Mocha Frost**
__Mushroom-Sausage Breakfast Bowl*

__Pumpkin Spice Oats*
__**Starbucks Spinach and Feta Breakfast Wrap**
__**Sunny Grape-Buckwheat Breakfast Bowl**
__**Sweet Delight Overnight Oat and Chia Pudding**

LUNCH AND DINNER

Hunger level _____

__**Chipotle Burrito Bowl**
__**Creamy-Crispy Tofu Salad**
__Curried Black Bean and Corn Burger over Quinoa Salad*
__**Feta-Mushroom Crab Cake over Basil-Olive Buckwheat**
__**Grilled Chicken and Sweet Potato Sandwich**
__Lemon-Salmon Tabbouleh*
__Outback Steakhouse 6-Ounce Victoria's Filet, Grilled Asparagus, and Baked Potato*
__**Oven-"Fried" Tofu Sticks with Creamy Peanut-Soy Dip**
__**Panera Bread Chicken Cobb with Avocado**

__Quinoa Enchiladas*
__**Rosemary Pork Tenderloin with Parmesan Potato Spears**
__Southwestern Salad with Cilantro Dressing*
__Spiced Turkey-Veggie-Quinoa Scramble/Wrap*
__Starbucks Hearty Veggie and Brown Rice Salad Bowl*
__**Sweet and Savory Brown Rice Salad with Chicken, Cheese, and Greens**
__Tomato, Onion, and Parmesan Salmon Frittata*
__Tuna Niçoise Salad*

__Tuna Tacos with Zucchini Slaw, Spicy Yogurt Sauce, and Salsa Brown Rice
__Turkey Sausage–Mushroom-Onion Stuffed Baked Potato with Roasted Cauliflower*

__Whole Grain Penne with Ricotta, Grape Tomatoes, and Broccoli

SNACKS (100 CALORIES)

Hunger level _____

__Asian Edamame and Carrot Salad*
__Chopped Apple, Feta, and Mint Salad
__Cumin–Black Bean Dip with Carrots*
__Frozen Banana–Almond Butter Sandwiches

__Mini Tomato-Chickpea Quesadilla
__Salmon and Corn Salad*
__Tomato-Parmesan Bites*
__Tuna and Chopped Olives with Lemon and Dried Dillweed

SNACKS (150 CALORIES)

Hunger level _____

__Apple Slices with Chia-Yogurt Drizzle
__Cauliflower Florets and Hummus*
__Chili-Spiced Turkey Avocado Roll-Ups*
__Cinnamon-Walnut Quinoa*

__Creamy Kale Salad*
__Crisp-Roasted Cinnamon Chickpeas
__Strawberry Ba-Nilla Snack Smoothie
__Whole Grain Crispbread with Almond Butter and Sliced Grapes

ADDITIONAL FOODS

NOTES

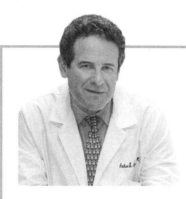

Sweet Inspiration

Arthur Agatston, MD

Be a sugar sleuth. It's important to remember that sugar isn't just found in the sugar bowl. It's added to a vast array of products from salad dressings and soups to tomato sauce and peanut butter, and found naturally in carbohydrate-rich foods like bread and potatoes.

Fiber matters! The more highly processed and lacking in fiber the foods you eat are, the more they can cause the swings in blood sugar that can lead to cravings for more refined sugars and starches. It's a vicious cycle. A substantial part of your diet should consist of nutrient-dense, high-fiber real foods—fruits, vegetables, and whole grains—that will keep you feeling satisfied longer and make you less likely to overeat.

Cut back gradually. Getting used to less sugar can be tough for some people, so I recommend that you start by eliminating the foods that are the biggest problems—soda and fruit drinks, candy, sweet bakery goods like cookies and muffins, and ice cream. It may take a few days for your body to adjust, but I guarantee that if you do so, your cravings for it will disappear.

Tap into the power of three. On special occasions, most people (including myself) want to enjoy a decadent dessert. For such times I recommend the South Beach Diet Three-Bite Rule: Have three bites and then put the dessert aside for a few minutes or pass your plate to a fellow diner or the busboy. You'll find that three bites of any dessert will satisfy you without triggering your desire to keep eating. Having a small piece of dark chocolate (at least 70 percent cacao) after a meal instead of dessert can also do the trick. Several studies have shown that eating dark chocolate in moderation can lower blood pressure (probably due to the beneficial effects of its polyphenols on blood vessel elasticity and bloodflow) and reduce levels of C-reactive protein (CRP) in the body, a powerful predictor of heart disease and type 2 diabetes. The flavonoids in dark chocolate and cocoa powder may also help protect against certain forms of cancer and diabetes.

ARTHUR AGATSTON, MD, is the medical director of Wellness and Prevention for Baptist Health South Florida and a clinical professor of medicine at the Florida International University Herbert Wertheim College of Medicine. He is the creator of the best-selling South Beach Diet book series. Most recently, he is the author of *The South Beach Diet Gluten Solution* and *The South Beach Diet Gluten Solution Cookbook.*

EAT THIS
Phase 2 Quick & Easy Meals

Have three meals and two snacks every day from the options below.

Breakfast Choices

Express on the Go

Along with the dining-out options in Phase 1, you may have for breakfast.

Starbucks Spinach and Feta Breakfast Wrap

Per serving: 290 calories, 19 g protein, 33 g carbohydrates, 6 g fiber, 4 g total sugar, 2 g added sugar (estimated), 10 g fat, 4 g saturated fat, 830 mg sodium

Breakfast Brown Rice Fritter

Whisk the egg and egg white with a pinch each of sea salt, black pepper, and garlic powder. Stir in the brown rice, sausage, onion, spinach, and mushrooms. Form into a fritter. In a medium skillet over medium-high heat, heat 1½ teaspoons olive oil. Cook the fritter for 6 minutes, turning once, or until browned.

Per serving: 297 calories, 17 g protein, 27 g carbohydrates, 2 g fiber, 2 g total sugar, 14 g fat, 3 g saturated fat, 314 mg sodium

Shopping list:

1 egg + 1 egg white

¼ cup cooked brown rice

1 link chicken sausage (such as Hormel Natural Choice Jalapeño Cheddar, Trader Joe's Spicy Italian, or Applegate Organics Fire Roasted Red Pepper)

2 tablespoons chopped onion

2 tablespoons chopped spinach

2 tablespoons chopped mushrooms

Creamy Mocha Frost

In a blender, combine the banana, milk, 1½ teaspoons unsweetened cocoa powder, ½ teaspoon instant coffee, almond butter, and tofu. Blend on high speed for 1 minute, or until smooth. Add 1 cup ice. Blend on high for 45 seconds, or until no ice chunks remain.

Per serving: 302 calories, 17 g protein, 44 g carbohydrates, 5 g fiber, 27 g total sugar, 9 g fat, 1.5 g saturated fat, 136 mg sodium

Shopping list:

1 very ripe banana

1 cup fat-free milk

2 teaspoons almond butter

¼ cup soft (not silken) tofu, drained

I had the Creamy Mocha Frost for breakfast. Delicious!
—Michelle

Sunny Grape-Buckwheat Breakfast Bowl

Stir ⅛ teaspoon ground cinnamon and 1 teaspoon warm water into the almond butter. Set aside. Stir the grapes into the buckwheat. Drizzle with the cinnamon–almond butter mixture. Serve with a coffee milk made by stirring 1 teaspoon instant coffee into the milk.

Shopping list:
1 tablespoon almond butter
½ cup halved red grapes
½ cup cooked buckwheat
1 cup fat-free milk, warmed

Per serving: 317 calories, 15 g protein, 46 g carbohydrates, 5 g fiber, 25 g total sugar, 10 g fat, 1 g saturated fat, 135 mg sodium

Sweet Delight Overnight Oat and Chia Pudding

Chop half of the apple. In a bowl, combine the milk, chia seeds, ⅛ teaspoon ground cinnamon, and oats. Add the chopped apple. Cover the mixture and refrigerate overnight. In the morning, chop the other half of the apple. Mix it with the walnuts and a pinch of cinnamon. Use as a topping for the oats.

Shopping list:
1 apple
¾ cup fat-free milk
1 teaspoon chia seeds
⅓ cup rolled oats
2 teaspoons chopped walnuts

Per serving: 293 calories, 14 g protein, 49 g carbohydrates, 8 g fiber, 24 g total sugar, 7 g fat, 1 g saturated fat, 100 mg sodium

FAQs for Phase 2

**Q: *Can I swap dried fruit or fruit juice for fresh fruit,
and eat canned fruit instead of fresh?***

A: No. While dried fruit contains all the fiber and nutrients of fresh,
it's extremely high in calories and sugar. For example, ½ cup of dried
apricot halves contains 157 calories and 35 grams of sugar, while
the same amount of fresh apricot halves packs 37 calories
and 7 grams of sugar. That's why this plan counts dried fruit as a
natural sweetener, like honey or maple syrup. In Phase 3, you'll
learn to use it as a Flavor Booster—just a bit packs a powerful
amount of sweetness!

Avoid fruit juice, too. It contains more sugar than fruit, and even
though that sugar is natural, it contributes calories. For instance,
an 8-ounce glass of orange juice has 112 calories, 21 grams of
sugar, and 0.5 gram of fiber. A medium navel orange has 69 calories,
12 grams of sugar, and 3 grams of fiber. The juice will be converted
into blood sugar more quickly than the orange will. Moreover, calories
that you drink simply don't fill you up. Liquids don't trigger your satiety
mechanism the same way whole foods do, and juice doesn't have the
critical fiber component that whole fruit offers.

As for canned fruit, I'd stick to fresh if possible. Canned fruit
packed in heavy or light syrup contains tons of sugar, while varieties
canned in fruit juice contain more calories and sugar than fresh or
frozen (unsweetened) fruit. Water-packed fruits are often sweetened
with artificial sweeteners, but if you can find a water-packed brand
that isn't, that's a fine choice.

Lunch and Dinner Choices

Sweet and Savory Brown Rice Salad with Chicken, Cheese, and Greens

Toss the arugula with the apple, sausage link, brown rice, 2 teaspoons olive oil, a pinch of garlic powder, and feta cheese.

Per serving: 450 calories, 25 g protein, 38 g carbohydrates, 4 g fiber, 11 g total sugar, 24 g fat, 9 g saturated fat, 931 mg sodium

Shopping list:

2 cups arugula

½ cup chopped apple

1 precooked chicken sausage link, chopped

½ cup cooked brown rice

¼ cup feta cheese

Express on the Go

Along with the dining-out options in Phase 1, you may have for lunch or dinner:

Chipotle Burrito Bowl

Order a burrito bowl with steak or chicken, black beans, fajita vegetables, roasted chili-corn salsa, fresh tomato salsa, and lettuce. Skip the rice and ask for extra beans.

Per serving: 435 calories, 42 g protein, 49 g carbohydrates, 17 g fiber, 11 g total sugar, <1 g added sugar (estimated), 10 g fat, 2 g saturated fat, 1,450 mg sodium

Panera Bread Chicken Cobb with Avocado

Ask for the Greek/Herb Vinaigrette dressing on the side and use half the dressing. Skip the side of bread.

Per serving: 470 calories, 38 g protein, 14 g carbohydrates, 6 g fiber, 2 g total sugar, 0 g added sugar, 30 g fat, 8 g saturated fat, 900 mg sodium

Creamy-Crispy Tofu Salad

Whisk together the yogurt, ⅛ teaspoon sea salt, ½ teaspoon mustard (your favorite variety), lemon juice, parsley, garlic, a pinch of black pepper, and avocado. Using a fork, stir the mixture into the tofu, pressing the dressing into the tofu thoroughly. Stir in the spinach. Spread the mixture onto the crispbreads *or* wrap. Top each crispbread with 1 tablespoon of bell pepper; if making a wrap, add all of the bell pepper to the salad.

Per serving: 457 calories, 20 g protein, 59 g carbohydrates, 12 g fiber, 7 g total sugar, 15 g fat, 2.5 g saturated fat, 447 mg sodium

Shopping list:

3 tablespoons low-fat plain yogurt

1 teaspoon lemon juice

1 teaspoon chopped fresh parsley

¼ teaspoon minced garlic

¼ avocado, mashed

¾ cup drained soft (not silken) tofu, crumbled

1 cup chopped baby spinach

4 whole grain crispbreads (such as Wasa brand) or 1 whole grain wrap (10″)

¼ cup chopped red bell pepper

Feta-Mushroom Crab Cake over Basil-Olive Buckwheat

Whisk ½ teaspoon mustard (your favorite variety) and the garlic with the egg white. Stir in the crab meat, mushrooms, and feta cheese. Gently stir in the bread crumbs. Form the mixture into a patty. In a medium skillet over medium-high heat, heat 1 teaspoon olive oil. Cook the cake for 8 minutes, turning once, or until cooked through and browned. Serve over the buckwheat mixed with ½ teaspoon olive oil, the basil, and the olives.

Per serving: 444 calories, 25 g protein, 36 g carbohydrates, 5 g fiber, 4 g total sugar, 23 g fat, 9 g saturated fat, 864 mg sodium

Shopping list:

¼ teaspoon chopped garlic

1 egg white

¼ cup drained canned crab meat

2 tablespoons finely chopped cremini mushrooms

2 tablespoons crumbled feta cheese

2 tablespoons whole grain bread crumbs (such as Ian's Whole Wheat Panko Bread Crumbs)

¾ cup cooked buckwheat

1 tablespoon chopped fresh basil

2 tablespoons chopped Greek olives

I made the Feta-Mushroom Crab Cake tonight. OMG. This is staying on the roster. Quick, easy, and super delicious. —Nora

Grilled Chicken and Sweet Potato Sandwich

In a medium skillet over medium-high heat, heat 1 teaspoon olive oil. Cook the kale, ⅛ teaspoon salt, and a pinch of black pepper, stirring frequently, for 4 minutes, or until the kale wilts. Using ½ teaspoon olive oil, warm the chicken breast. Slice the sweet potato in half. On one half of the potato, place the chicken, sun-dried tomato, feta cheese, and the kale. Top with the other half of the potato to form a sandwich.

Per serving: 428 calories, 35 g protein, 45 g carbohydrates, 8 g fiber, 13 g total sugar, 13 g fat, 3 g saturated fat, 557 mg sodium

Shopping list:

- **1 cup chopped kale**
- **1 slice (3 ounces) roasted skinless chicken breast**
- **1 sweet potato, baked**
- **1 tablespoon chopped sun-dried tomato**
- **1 tablespoon crumbled feta cheese**

Without sugar, I feel free. I no longer feel as if I am being controlled by my appetite. I love feeling content when I eat, and food tastes so much better. —Robyn

Oven-"Fried" Tofu Sticks and Eggplant with Creamy Peanut-Soy Dip

Preheat the oven to 425°F. Toss the eggplant with 1 teaspoon olive oil, a pinch of salt, and ½ teaspoon of the minced garlic. Mix the bread crumbs with ¼ teaspoon each garlic powder, smoked paprika, salt, black pepper, and chili powder. In a separate dish, whisk the egg. Slice the tofu into 4 sticks, placing each on a paper towel to absorb excess moisture. Working with 1 stick at a time, dip it into the egg, coating all sides, and then into the bread crumb mixture. Do the same with the eggplant. Place the coated sticks and eggplant on a baking sheet coated with cooking spray and bake for 25 minutes, turning once, or until crispy and golden on the outside. Serve with a dip made by whisking the yogurt with the soy sauce, remaining ¼ teaspoon garlic, and peanut butter.

Per serving: 442 calories, 26 g protein, 29 g carbohydrates, 6 g fiber, 10 g total sugar, 27 g fat, 5 g saturated fat, 772 mg sodium

Shopping list:

1 cup cubed eggplant

¾ teaspoon minced garlic

⅓ cup whole grain bread crumbs

1 egg

4.5 ounces (about ⅓ block) extra-firm tofu, drained

2 tablespoons low-fat plain yogurt

1 teaspoon reduced-sodium soy sauce

1 teaspoon peanut butter (such as Smucker's, Santa Cruz, Maranatha, or Trader Joe's)

Rosemary Pork Tenderloin with Parmesan Potato Spears

Preheat the oven to 425°F. Cut the potatoes into wedges, spray with cooking spray, and toss with the Parmesan cheese. Bake for 45 minutes, turning once, or until golden on the outside and soft inside. Meanwhile, toss the grapes and green beans with 1 teaspoon olive oil and ⅛ teaspoon salt and bake for 25 minutes, or until the grapes start to shrivel and the beans soften. Rub the pork tenderloin with a pinch each of salt and black pepper and ⅛ teaspoon dried rosemary and bake for 12 minutes, or until it reaches an internal temperature of 160°F and the juices run clear. Toss the grapes and beans with the lemon juice and garlic and serve over the pork with the potatoes on the side.

Per serving: 447 calories, 34 g protein, 58 g carbohydrates, 9 g fiber, 21 g total sugar, 10 g fat, 3 g saturated fat, 532 mg sodium

Shopping list:

2 small yellow potatoes

2 tablespoons grated Parmesan cheese

¾ cup red grapes

1 cup green beans

4 ounces pork tenderloin

½ teaspoon lemon juice

¼ teaspoon minced garlic

Tuna Tacos with Zucchini Slaw, Spicy Yogurt Sauce, and Salsa Brown Rice

Whisk the yogurt with a pinch each of salt, cumin, and ground red pepper. Place half the tuna in the center of each corn tortilla. Top each with half the zucchini and drizzle with half the yogurt sauce. Serve with the rice mixed with the salsa.

Per serving: 462 calories, 31 g protein, 61 g carbohydrates, 7 g fiber, 5 g total sugar, 10 g fat, 2 g saturated fat, 519 mg sodium

Shopping list:

2 tablespoons low-fat plain yogurt

2½ tablespoons drained, flaked oil-packed tuna

2 corn tortillas (6" diameter) (such as Food for Life Sprouted Corn Tortillas or La Tortilla Factory Yellow Corn Tortillas)

¼ cup grated zucchini

¾ cup cooked brown rice

2 tablespoons salsa

Whole Grain Penne with Ricotta, Grape Tomatoes, and Broccoli

Cook the penne according to package directions, but add the broccoli florets for the last 5 minutes of cooking time. Once drained, return the pasta and broccoli to the pan; stir in the ricotta cheese, a pinch of black pepper, and the tomatoes. Stir gently to coat the pasta with the cheese.

Per serving: 443 calories, 26 g protein, 65 g carbohydrates, 8 g fiber, 4 g total sugar, 11 g fat, 6 g saturated fat, 179 mg sodium

Shopping list:

⅔ cup whole grain penne

½ cup broccoli florets

½ cup part-skim ricotta cheese

½ cup halved grape tomatoes

Fruit and Protein Combos

For a quick 100-calorie snack, pick one item from each of the two charts below. None of these foods contain any added sugar.

Fruit

Serving of Fruit	Calories	Carbs (g)	Fiber (g)	Sugar (g)
Apple, 1 cup sliced	57	15	3	11
Banana, ½ large	61	16	2	8
Blackberries, 1 cup	62	14	8	7
Blueberries, ¾ cup	63	16	3	11
Cherries, 12	62	15	2	13
Clementines, 2	70	18	3	14
Figs (fresh), 2	74	19	3	16
Grapefruit, 1 large	53	13	2	12
Grapes, 20	68	18	<1	15
Guava, 2	74	16	6	10
Kiwifruit, ½ cup sliced	55	13	3	8
Mango, ½ cup chunks	50	12	1	11
Melon, 1 cup chunks	61	15	1	14
Orange, 1 medium	65	16	3	13
Papaya, 1 cup chunks	62	16	3	11
Peach, 1 medium	58	14	2	13
Pear, ¾ cup slices	60	16	3	10
Pineapple, 1 cup chunks	62	16	2	12
Plums, 2 medium	61	15	2	13
Raspberries, 1 cup	64	15	8	5
Starfruit, 1 cup sliced	33	7	3	4
Strawberries, 1 cup sliced	53	12	4	8
Tangerine, 1 medium	47	12	2	9
Watermelon, 1 cup balls	37	9	<1	8

Fruit contains 1 gram or less of protein and fat and minimal sodium.

Protein Snacks

Serving of Protein	Calories	Protein (g)	Carbs (g)	Fiber (g)	Sugar (g)	Fat (g)	Saturated Fat (g)	Sodium (mg)
Almond butter, ½ Tbsp	49	2	2	<1	<1	4	<1	18
Almonds, 6	41	2	2	<1	<1	4	<1	0
Cashews, 4	49	1	3	<1	<1	4	1	1
Cheddar cheese, low-fat, 1 oz	48	7	1	0	<1	2	1	171
Cottage cheese, low-fat, ¼ cup	41	7	2	0	2	<1	<1	229
Peanut butter, ½ Tbsp	47	2	2	<1	<1	4	<1	37
Pistachios, 10	40	1	2	<1	<1	3	<1	0
Ricotta, part-skim, ⅛ cup	39	3	2	0	<1	2	1	35
Roast beef, deli, 3 slices	48	7	1	0	0	1	<1	366
Swiss cheese, low-fat, 1 oz	48	8	1	0	<1	1	<1	73
Turkey, deli, 2 slices	55	13	0	<1	2	<1	<1	432
Walnuts, 3 halves	46	1	1	<1	<1	5	<1	0
Yogurt, Greek, 0% plain, ¼ cup	50	9	3	0	3	<1	<1	31
Yogurt, regular, fat-free plain, ⅓ cup	46	5	6	0	6	<1	<1	63

Snack Choices (1 per Day—100 Calories)

Chopped Apple, Feta, and Mint Salad

Chop the apple and toss it with the mint, feta cheese, and 1 teaspoon olive oil.

Per serving: 100 calories, 1 g protein, 10 g carbohydrates, 2 g fiber, 8 g total sugar, 6 g fat, 2 g saturated fat, 102 mg sodium

Shopping list:
½ apple
1 teaspoon chopped fresh mint
1 tablespoon crumbled feta cheese

Frozen Banana–Almond Butter Sandwiches

Slice the banana into 6 thin slices, widthwise. Spread 3 slices with ½ teaspoon of the almond butter. Top each with another banana slice to form a sandwich. Freeze for an hour or overnight.

Per serving: 102 calories, 2 g protein, 15 g carbohydrates, 2 g fiber, 8 g total sugar, 5 g fat, <1 g saturated fat, 115 mg sodium

Shopping list:
½ banana
1½ teaspoons almond butter

Casting around for fruit for the last snack of the day, I hit on the organic mango chunks in my freezer. Ate several chunks frozen, straight out of the bag. Ambrosia! Creamy, fruity, sweet, and cold. I heartily recommend them as a decadent frozen treat! –Jean

Mini Tomato-Chickpea Quesadilla

Spread the chickpeas onto the corn tortilla. Sprinkle with the tomato and mozzarella cheese. Microwave on medium power for 45 seconds, or until the cheese melts. Fold in half and top with the salsa.

Per serving: 114 calories, 6 g protein, 17 g carbohydrates, 2 g fiber, 1 g total sugar, 3 g fat, 1.5 g saturated fat, 148 mg sodium

Shopping list:

2 tablespoons mashed chickpeas

1 corn tortilla (6″ diameter)

2 tablespoons chopped tomato

1½ tablespoons shredded part-skim mozzarella cheese

2 teaspoons salsa

Tuna and Chopped Olives with Lemon and Dried Dillweed

Toss the tuna with the olive, lemon juice, and ⅛ teaspoon dried dillweed.

Per serving: 108 calories, 15 g protein, <1 g carbohydrates, <1 g fiber, <1 g total sugar, 5 g fat, <1 g saturated fat, 246 mg sodium

Shopping list:

¼ cup drained and flaked oil-packed tuna

1 Greek olive, chopped

½ teaspoon lemon juice

Snack Choices (1 per Day—150 Calories)

Apple Slices with Chia-Yogurt Drizzle

Stir the chia seeds and ¼ teaspoon vanilla extract into the yogurt. Drizzle over the apple or blueberries.

Per serving: 145 calories, 4 g protein, 26 g carbs, 7 g fiber, 17 g total sugar, 4 g fat, <1 g saturated fat, 34 mg sodium

Shopping list:

2 teaspoons chia seeds

3 tablespoons low-fat plain yogurt

1 apple, sliced, or 1 cup blueberries

Crisp-Roasted Cinnamon Chickpeas

Preheat the oven to 425°F. Allow the chickpeas to dry on a paper towel. Once the excess water is absorbed, toss the chickpeas with 1 teaspoon olive oil. Toss again with ¼ teaspoon ground cinnamon. Bake for 20 minutes, stirring several times, or until golden and crunchy.

Per serving: 146 calories, 5 g protein, 18 g carbohydrates, <1 g fiber, <1 g total sugar, 6 g fat, <1 g saturated fat, 161 mg sodium

Shopping list:

½ cup canned chickpeas, rinsed and drained

Strawberry Ba-Nilla Snack Smoothie

In a blender, combine the milk, straw-berries, banana, and ¼ teaspoon vanilla extract. Blend on high for 1 minute, or until smooth. Add 3 ice cubes and blend again for 45 seconds, or until no ice chunks remain.

Per serving: 135 calories, 7 g protein, 27 g carbohydrates, 3 g fiber, 19 g total sugar, <1 g fat, <1 g saturated fat, 90 mg sodium

Shopping list:
¾ cup fat-free milk
4 large strawberries
½ very ripe banana

Whole Grain Crispbread with Almond Butter and Sliced Grapes

Spread the almond butter onto the crispbread. Top with the grapes.

Per serving: 162 calories, 3 g protein, 18 g carbohydrates, 4 g fiber, 4 g total sugar, 0 g fat, <1 g saturated fat, 52 mg sodium

Shopping list:
1 tablespoon almond butter
1 whole grain crispbread
4 grapes, sliced into thirds

Sweet Dreams!
Sleepy Breathing

If your brain refuses to shut off at night, use "breathwork" to calm it. Long, slow abdominal breathing can reduce anxiety and arousal, according to a small Harvard study. Volunteers who used yoga breathing techniques to treat insomnia reported improvements in the quality and quantity of their sleep.

To sleep better tonight, try the 4-7-8 breath exercise. Resting your tongue on the roof of your mouth, just behind your upper teeth (your mouth should be slightly open), exhale deeply. Close your mouth and inhale through your nose for 4 counts. Hold your breath for 7 counts. Then exhale while mentally counting to 8. Repeat the cycle three more times.

YOU GOT THIS
Managing Stress and Cravings in Phase 2

Now that you're eating sugar again, in fruit, your hankering for sweets should be history, or nearly so. Still, stress or intense emotions have a way of triggering cravings, which can pull you back into sugar's snare. To avoid being blindsided, stay mindful as you eat and cool stress as soon as it flares. You've built up quite an array of coping strategies, but here are two more tools for your toolbox.

Cravings Crusher: Switch to Sugar-Free Volunteering

Luckily, I don't regularly bake goodies for soccer games, school fairs, or other events. I strongly suspect that if I did, more cookie dough would end up in my mouth than on the baking sheets! While cravings can come out of nowhere, they can also be triggered by the sight and smell of particular foods, and handling the ingredients for sweet treats–even if they're meant for someone else–can lead sugar straight back to your mouth, and belly.

If you do a lot of "volunteer feeding" and sugar cravings are an issue for you, I recommend that you ask or sign up for another way to volunteer your services instead. For example, if you typically prepare or hand out sugary snacks and drinks to your child's sports team, hand out bottles of water instead. Or if you always bake sweets for school dances or the annual church carnival, volunteer to chaperone or take tickets instead.

Part of being sugar smart is knowing your weaknesses, accepting them, loving yourself anyway–and removing yourself from situations that get your sweet buds all hot and tingly. It's more than okay to remove yourself from those situations. In fact, it's essential to your health and well-being.

Sweet Freedom Strategy: Cool Conflict Hawaiian-Style

In general, I have a positive view of conflict. Time and again, I've seen that working through disagreements in a positive way, rather than avoiding them, fosters growth. Of course, conflict can be uncomfortable. And because I'm only human, there have been times when I chose the gelato method of conflict resolution. Each time, that path led to resentment, stress, and way too much sugar and carbs.

So when I read about *ho'oponopono* (pronounced "ho-o-pono-pono"), my antennae went up. Researchers who have examined this ancient Hawaiian method of conflict resolution, forgiveness, and peacemaking have found that it can help people manage stress and find peace. (This technique has even been found to reduce blood pressure!)

The word *ho'oponopono* comes from *ho'o* ("to make") and *pono* ("right"). You can practice this method all by yourself, and it can help "make things right" in a way that sugar and carbs only pretend to.

You can use *ho'oponopono* to forgive others (spouse, kids, parents, boss, coworker, surly cashier) or yourself, and you can do it alone. All you need do is say, silently or out loud:

I'm sorry.
Please forgive me.
I love you.
Thank you.

Repeat until you feel at peace. Yes, it's that simple. And powerful.

Maria Kita

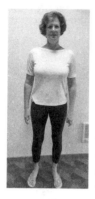

Maria Kita looks like the picture of health. She could even be on the cover of *Prevention* magazine. But she was keeping a dirty little secret. "I would hide bags of my favorite sweet and salty treats from my family so no one else would eat them," says Maria, a nurse and yoga instructor. "While I'd be eating a meal, I was thinking about the snacks that I'd have later!" Maria's snacking usually started with something crunchy and salty, like chips or cheese curls, followed by a sweet like chocolate. When she tried to deprive herself, it usually backfired. "I'd eat more and feel even worse."

In her twenties, thirties, and forties, Maria was able to eat what she wanted without worrying about gaining weight. But that changed once she hit her fifties. "My clothes were getting too tight, and I had to buy new ones in larger sizes," says Maria. With menopause nearing and the threat of packing on more pounds, Maria was ready to make some changes.

No more Pasta Roni for lunch! "I've pretty much cut out all processed foods," she says. And no more "chipping out," as her husband would call it, when she'd have her hand in a bag of cheese curls or chips as she watched TV or was on the computer.

Instead, Maria's eating protein-packed meals that are filling and provide her with the stamina she needs for her 3:15 a.m. wake-up calls. She's traded the cereal bars that she used to eat on her way into the hospital for Tomato-Parmesan Bites or tuna in a pita. "They're harder to eat and messier, but I'm less hungry later." And she has more energy. "I used to nap in the afternoon, but I don't have that urge anymore," she says. "I get more done."

When Maria has chosen to indulge, like at her mom's birthday party, she's been surprised at how satisfied she is with only a taste. "I used to laugh at models who said, 'Oh, you can have dessert—just have one bite.' But I totally understand now. I don't have to deprive myself. I can have a bite or two and my body just smiles and says, 'I'm happy now.'"

5.3
POUNDS LOST

AGE:
52

ALL-OVER INCHES LOST:
5

SUGAR SMART WISDOM:
"Turn mundane things into something special. Pour seltzer into a pretty glass and add a wedge of lime. It's almost as satisfying as a gin and tonic."

Days 12 to 16: Phase 3
Sugar, Naturally

PHASE 3 GOALS: To learn to use small amounts of five intensely sweet, all-natural sugars to add a touch of welcome sweetness to meals and snacks.

PHASE 3 BENEFITS: By Day 16, I hope, you're in the swing of the plan. After more than 2 weeks of savoring only whole foods, you've likely lost much of your longing for sweets and refined carbs and gained a new appreciation for flavor. While you may still experience occasional sugar cravings, you're more aware of how to manage or even prevent them. You should also notice a significant improvement in mood, sleep, and energy.

In this phase, you'll be dipping into pure honey and maple syrup, along with three other intense natural sweeteners: 100 percent fruit spread, dried fruit, and fruit juice. But as you'll see (and taste!), these sweeteners are used as *ingredients*, to make healthy meals more enjoyable. So you won't drink fruit juice; you'll cook with it. And you won't nosh dried fruit by the handful; you'll add small amounts to boost the flavor of tasty, healthy whole foods.

You'll savor one meal that contains these sweeteners per day. The maximum amounts:

- 1 teaspoon of honey *or* maple syrup
- 2 teaspoons of 100 percent fruit spread
- 2 to 3 tablespoons of dried fruit
- $\frac{1}{4}$ cup (or less) of fruit juice

While these amounts may seem small, they're all your now exquisitely sensitive taste buds need. Besides, these small amounts keep calories in check (these natural sweeteners are calorie-dense) and won't stir up your sugar cravings.

Because your bread options expand in this phase, you'll be getting added sugar in those, too. Want a whole grain English muffin? You got it. Ditto for sliced bread, rolls, and bagels (small ones). We've set a sugar content limit of 2 grams per slice of bread, English muffin, or burger bun/roll and 6 grams or less per bagel. (Bagels tend to contain more sugar because the sugar helps the chewy crust form during cooking.)

I recommend choosing a dense, seed-caught-in-your-back-tooth bread. (I usually buy breads made by the Food for Life Baking Company. Available in most supermarkets' organic sections, they come in a variety of forms–breads, buns, pocket breads, English muffins, tortillas–and most contain no added sugar. The slices are sturdy enough to enjoy as an open-face sandwich, and they toast up deliciously.)

Even so, stick to having processed grain products no more than once a day. Between the natural sweeteners and the added sugar in bread products, you could be taking in 2 teaspoons of added sugar a day in this phase, depending on what you choose to eat.

DO THIS
Phase 3 Strategies

- Have breakfast every morning.
- Mix and match the lunch and dinner options. You can keep eating any of the Phase 1 or Phase 2 quick and easy meals, as well as incorporate the new options in this phase.
- Remember that you have the option of eating one daily serving of a processed whole wheat or whole grain product, including pasta and bread. I stress the word *option*–if you don't miss them, don't eat them!
- Include one daily meal or snack that contains a natural sweetener, if you like. Like processed grain products, natural sweeteners are optional.
- Have fruit up to three times a day.
- Don't forget to snack!
- Avoid the following foods: white flour and products made with it, white rice, and fruit juice as a beverage.
- Set your daily intention.

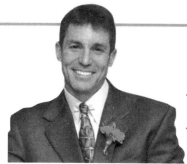

Sweet Inspiration

David L. Katz, MD, MPH

Make sugar do double duty. Enjoy sugar only in foods that really matter to you and that are also nutritious. Dark chocolate is a good example—it's good for you overall, but it certainly does contain added sugar.

Reboot your "sweet buds." Sweet is the only taste preference we're born with—it leads us to our mother's milk. The excess of sugar in modern food is a potent goad to appetite, exploiting this all-but-universal preference. But taste buds can be rehabilitated quite readily. The less sugar you eat in general, the less you need to feel satisfied and the less you tend to want. Simply by removing the Stealth Sugars in foods like jarred pasta sauces and salad dressings, you will likely start to prefer your food less sweet. Once you eliminate foods that contain Stealth Sugars, you can move on to beverages and desserts, where the sugar is more apparent.

Pick flavor over sugar. I prefer my desserts minimally sweetened. For example, when my wife bakes, she uses less than half the sugar a standard recipe calls for. I like dried fruit but not with added sugar. I don't understand how anyone would even think to sprinkle sugar over berries; they are plenty sweet enough direct from nature.

Learn to love foods that love you back. To keep my own sugar intake in check, I eat mostly natural, wholesome foods, getting intrinsic sugar in fruits and dairy foods. I don't drink soda, and I avoid eating foods that contain those Stealth Sugars. On any given day, I take in around 25 grams of added sugar or less, usually in dark chocolate, breakfast cereal, and, occasionally, my wife's cookies. We can all learn to love foods that love us back—we just have to get used to them as the norm. My family and I have done just that.

DAVID KATZ, MD, MPH, is the director of Yale University's Prevention Research Center, a clinical instructor in medicine at the Yale School of Medicine, editor-in-chief of the journal *Childhood Obesity*, founder and president of the nonprofit Turn the Tide Foundation, and medical director for the Integrative Medicine Center at Griffin Hospital in Derby, Connecticut. Most recently, he is the author of *Disease Proof: The Remarkable Truth about What Makes Us Well.*

DAILY FOOD LOG

PHASE 3

Date:

Today's intention:

Place an X next to the meals and snacks you ate today. You can mix and match your meals and snacks from Phases 1, 2, and 3. Boldface indicates an option added in this phase; an asterisk denotes a recipe that can be found in Chapters 7 or 8.

BREAKFAST

Hunger level _____

__**Banana-Ricotta Pancakes**
__Basil-Mozzarella Pancakes*
__Breakfast Brown Rice Fritter*
__**Breakfast Tostada**
__Cinnamon-Vanilla Egg White Crepes with Almond Butter Cream*
__Creamy Mocha Frost*
__**Deviled Egg Breakfast Sandwich**
__**Kiwi-Strawberry Muesli Parfait**

__**Loaded Toast**
__Mushroom-Sausage Breakfast Bowl*
__Pumpkin Spice Oats*
__Starbucks Spinach and Feta Breakfast Wrap*
__Sunny Grape-Buckwheat Breakfast Bowl*
__Sweet Delight Overnight Oat and Chia Pudding*

LUNCH AND DINNER

Hunger level _____

__**California Roast Beef Pita Sandwich**
__**Carrot Slaw with Edamame**
__**Cheddar Turkey Burger with Broccoli Slaw**
__**Chicken Sausage, Cabbage, and Kidney Bean Sauté**
__**Chicken Sausage with 'Kraut, Served with Carrot Fries**
__Chipotle Burrito Bowl*
__Creamy-Crispy Tofu Salad*
__Curried Black Bean and Corn Burger over Quinoa Salad*

__Feta-Mushroom Crab Cake over Basil-Olive Buckwheat*
__**Frozen Meal: Artisan Bistro Grass-Fed Beef with Mushroom Sauce**
__Grilled Chicken and Sweet Potato Sandwich*
__**Hearty Spinach Salad Vinaigrette with Steak, Strawberries, White Beans, and Pistachios**
__Lemon-Salmon Tabbouleh*
__Outback Steakhouse 6-Ounce Victoria's Filet, Grilled Asparagus, and Baked Potato*

(continued)

DAILY FOOD LOG (cont.)

__Oven-"Fried" Tofu Sticks with Creamy Peanut-Soy Dip*

__Panera Bread Chicken Cobb with Avocado*

__**Pepper Stuffed with Turkey, Wild Rice, and Pistachios**

__**Pork Chop with Maple Carrots and Wild Rice Pilaf**

__Quinoa Enchiladas*

__Rosemary Pork Tenderloin with Parmesan Potato Spears*

__Southwestern Salad with Cilantro Dressing*

__Spiced Turkey-Veggie-Quinoa Scramble/Wrap*

__Starbucks Hearty Veggie and Brown Rice Salad Bowl*

__**Steak with Strawberry Compote, Roasted Potatoes, and Roasted Garlic Broccoli**

__Sweet and Savory Brown Rice Salad with Chicken, Cheese, and Greens*

__Tomato, Onion, and Parmesan Salmon Frittata*

__Tuna Niçoise Salad*

__Tuna Tacos with Zucchini Slaw, Spicy Yogurt Sauce, and Salsa Brown Rice*

__Turkey Sausage–Mushroom-Onion Stuffed Baked Potato with Roasted Cauliflower*

__**Veggie Burger Wrap with Hummus and Avocado with Chipotle Kale Chips**

__Whole Grain Penne with Ricotta, Grape Tomatoes, and Broccoli*

SNACKS (100 CALORIES)

Hunger level _____

__Asian Edamame and Carrot Salad*

__**Basic Fruit and Protein**

__Chopped Apple, Feta, and Mint Salad*

__**Cocoa-Coconut Sliced Banana**

__**Creamy Avocado-Bean Wedge with Lemon**

__Cumin–Black Bean Dip with Carrots*

__Frozen Banana–Almond Butter Sandwiches*

__Mini Tomato-Chickpea Quesadilla*

__**Pepper Slices and Chunky Yogurt-Salsa Dip**

__**Pistachio-Ginger Kiwi Boats**

__Salmon and Corn Salad*

__Tomato-Parmesan Bites*

__Tuna and Chopped Olives with Lemon and Dried Dillweed*

SNACKS (150 CALORIES)

Hunger level _____

__Apple Slices with Chia-Yogurt Drizzle*

__**Banana-Strawberry Muesli**

__Cauliflower Florets and Hummus*

__Chili-Spiced Turkey Avocado Roll-Ups*

__Cinnamon-Walnut Quinoa*

__**Creamy-Fruity Ricotta with Honey**

__Creamy Kale Salad*

__Crisp-Roasted Cinnamon Chickpeas*

__**Green Tea–Cucumber Smoothie**

__**South of the Border English Muffin**

__Strawberry Ba-Nilla Snack
  Smoothie*

__**Strawberry Spice Boats**

__Whole Grain Crispbread with
  Almond Butter and Sliced Grapes*

ADDITIONAL FOODS

NOTES

SHOP THIS

Choose your meals and customize your shopping list. Each recipe is a single serving. If you're cooking for two or more people, multiply the ingredient quantities by the number of servings you want to make.

EAT THIS
Phase 3 Quick & Easy Meals

Have three meals and two snacks every day from the options below.

Breakfast Choices

Banana-Ricotta Pancakes

In a bowl, mix together the egg white, ricotta cheese, milk, oats, and banana. Coat a medium skillet with cooking spray and heat it over medium heat. Pour in the batter, forming 2 pancakes, and cook for 8 minutes, turning once, or until golden. Top with the maple syrup and coconut.

Per serving: 309 calories, 16 g protein, 46 g carbohydrates, 4 g fiber, 17 g total sugar, 8 g fat, 4 g saturated fat, 152 mg sodium

Shopping list:

1 egg white

¼ cup part-skim ricotta cheese

2 tablespoons fat-free milk

⅓ cup rolled oats

½ very ripe banana, mashed

2 teaspoons maple syrup

1 teaspoon unsweetened shredded coconut

Breakfast Tostada

Coat the tortillas with cooking spray. In a large skillet over medium heat, heat the tortillas for 4 minutes, turning once, or until the edges start to crisp. Remove from the skillet. Add ½ teaspoon olive oil and increase the heat to medium-high. Cook the egg and egg whites for 5 minutes, or until cooked to desired doneness. Sprinkle the eggs with a pinch of salt and black pepper. Place half of the eggs on each tortilla. Top each with half the avocado and 1 tablespoon chunky salsa.

Per serving: 292 calories, 17 g protein, 26 g carbohydrates, 6 g fiber, 2 g total sugar, 14 g fat, 3 g saturated fat, 393 mg sodium

Shopping list:

2 corn tortillas (6″ diameter) (such as Food for Life Sprouted Corn Tortillas or La Tortilla Factory Sonoma Yellow Corn Organic Tortillas)

1 egg + 2 egg whites, whisked

¼ avocado, finely chopped

2 tablespoons chunky salsa

Deviled Egg Breakfast Sandwich

In a bowl, using a fork, mash the egg and egg white. Mix in the hummus, pickle relish, and a pinch of paprika. Place the mixture on the toasted bottom half of the whole grain English muffin. Top with 1 slice tomato and the other half of the muffin.

Per serving: 285 calories, 17 g protein, 36 g carbohydrates, 6 g fiber, 8 g total sugar, 9 g fat, 2 g saturated fat, 479 mg sodium

Shopping list:

1 egg + 1 egg white, hard-cooked

2 tablespoons hummus

1 teaspoon sweet pickle relish

1 whole grain English muffin (such as Thomas' 100% Whole Wheat English Muffin or Trader Joe's Whole Wheat British Muffins)

1 slice tomato

Kiwi-Strawberry Muesli Parfait

In a bowl, whisk together the yogurt, maple syrup, and ¼ teaspoon vanilla extract. Layer half the mixture into a parfait glass or tall clear drinking glass. Top with half the oats, half the chopped kiwifruit, and half the chopped strawberries. Add the remaining yogurt. Top with a second layer of oats and fruit.

Per serving: 296 calories, 13 g protein, 52 g carbohydrates, 7 g fiber, 25 g total sugar, 5 g fat, 2 g saturated fat, 110 mg sodium

Shopping list:
⅔ cup low-fat plain yogurt
1 teaspoon maple syrup
6 tablespoons rolled oats
1 kiwifruit, peeled and chopped
4 large strawberries, chopped

Loaded Toast

Spread the peanut butter onto the toast. Top with the strawberries, pistachios, and honey. Serve with the milk topped with ground cinnamon.

Per serving: 294 calories, 14 g protein, 43 g carbohydrates, 6 g fiber, 24 g total sugar, 8 g fat, 2 g saturated fat, 236 mg sodium

Shopping list:
2 teaspoons peanut butter
1 slice whole grain bread, toasted
2 large strawberries, sliced
1 teaspoon chopped pistachios
1 teaspoon honey
1 cup fat-free milk, warmed

Pancakes: Guilt-Free Goodness

I can admit it: I love pancakes. In fact, I make them once or twice a week for my kids' breakfast and scarf a few myself. I can enjoy them right along with my kids because my pancakes are healthier than they taste—and they taste delicious.

I use whole wheat flour, rather than white flour. (We love our whole wheat 'cakes, but you might try a blend of whole wheat and almond or coconut flours, which have a lighter texture.) For sweetness, I add 1 or 2 mashed bananas, cinnamon, and a ton of vanilla extract. The result: satisfying, stick-to-your-ribs pancakes that are naturally sweet. Occasionally, as a treat, we top them with maple syrup—just a drizzle. When you splurge on the real deal, from Vermont, you really don't need more than that!

The Sugar Smart Express Skinny on Honey

Good to know: The thick, delectable liquid we spoon into tea or spread on toast starts as nectar from flowers, including clover, buckwheat, and orange blossoms. Hardworking honeybees break down that nectar into simple sugars. Packed into honeycombs and fanned constantly by bee wings, the nectar evaporates. Presto! Honey. Depending on the type of nectar that bees collect, honey can be nearly colorless or dark amber, and its taste delicate or robust. As a general rule, however, the lighter the honey, the milder the flavor.

Sweet 'n' healthy: Honey contains an estimated 180 different substances—proteins, enzymes, amino acids, minerals, vitamins, phytochemicals—that may account for its health-promoting effects. For example, gram for gram, honey is as rich in antioxidants as some fruits and veggies. Of course, we eat honey in small quantities (at least we should because it's calorie dense). But even small amounts may offer some protection against cancer and promote heart health. In test tube studies, honey—the darker the better—slows the oxidation of LDL ("bad") cholesterol in human blood. Oxidized LDLs are the foundation of dangerous plaque deposits in blood vessel walls that can lead to heart attack and stroke.

Get the best: Clover honey is the variety easiest to find in most supermarkets. But you can do better. Buckwheat honey contains eight times the antioxidant punch of the clover variety. Sunflower honey boasts three times as many antioxidants, followed by tupelo honey, with twice the antioxidant power.

But why buy at the supermarket? On Saturday mornings, my kids and I head to the farmers' market, where we love taste-testing different local honeys. They usually opt for mellow flavors, while I lean toward the rich, dark varieties.

Store it right: Store your honey at room temperature (your kitchen counter or pantry shelf is ideal). It will keep indefinitely. If it crystallizes, just place the jar in warm water and it will clear.

Lunch and Dinner Choices

California Roast Beef Pita Sandwich

Mash the avocado with a fork. Add a pinch of red-pepper flakes. Slice the pita in half and stuff each half with the avocado mixture. Add the onion, tomatoes, arugula, and roast beef.

Per serving: 450 calories, 33 g protein, 54 g carbohydrates, 10 g fiber, 3 g total sugar, 14 g fat, 3 g saturated fat, 583 mg sodium

Shopping list:

⅓ avocado

1 whole grain pita (6")
(such as Ezekiel 4:9
Whole Grain Pocket Bread)

1 tablespoon chopped onion

¼ cup halved grape tomatoes

1 cup arugula

3 thin slices reduced-sodium lean
roast beef (such as Boar's Head)

Express on the Go

Along with the dining-out options in Phases 1 and 2, you may have this healthy frozen meal.

Artisan Bistro Grass-Fed Beef with Mushroom Sauce

Serve with a side of 2 cups microwaved frozen or fresh broccoli topped with 1½ tablespoons sliced almonds and 1 teaspoon lemon juice.

Per serving: 468 calories, 30 g protein, 102 g carbohydrates, 6 g fiber, 6 g total sugar, 2 g added sugar (estimated), 20 g fat, 4 g saturated fat, 619 mg sodium

Want a different frozen meal? Follow these guidelines. Aim for:

300 to 450 calories (If the frozen meal is under 425 calories, add 1½ to 2 cups of veggies with 2 teaspoons olive oil or butter.)

At least 8 grams of protein

At least 4 grams of fiber

No more than 700 milligrams of sodium

No added sugars or artificial sweeteners

Carrot Slaw with Edamame

In a bowl, whisk together 1 table-spoon toasted sesame oil, the garlic, ginger, 1 teaspoon rice vinegar, orange juice, and 2½ teaspoons reduced-sodium soy sauce. In another bowl, toss together the edamame, rice, and carrot. Pour the dressing over the veggie mixture; toss to coat. Sprinkle with 1 tablespoon sesame seeds.

Per serving: 455 calories, 22 g protein, 46 g carbohydrates, 13 g fiber, 7 g total sugar, 22 g fat, 3 g saturated fat, 404 mg sodium

Shopping list:

¼ teaspoon minced garlic

¼ teaspoon minced fresh ginger

2 teaspoons orange juice

1 cup shelled edamame

½ cup cooked wild rice

½ cup shredded carrot

Cheddar Turkey Burger with Broccoli Slaw

Mix the yogurt with 1 teaspoon apple cider vinegar, 1 teaspoon finely chopped onion, ⅛ teaspoon sea salt, and a pinch of paprika. Stir dressing into ¼ cup shredded broccoli; set aside. Cook the turkey burger accord-ing to instructions. Place the burger on the bun and top with the cheese and the broccoli slaw. Serve with the orange.

Per serving: 454 calories, 34 g protein, 33 g carbohydrates, 5 g fiber, 12 g total sugar, 20 g fat, 9 g saturated fat, 540 mg sodium

Shopping list:

1½ tablespoons low-fat plain yogurt

1 teaspoon finely chopped onion

¼ cup shredded broccoli

1 lean 4-ounce turkey burger (such as an Applegate Organic Turkey Burger)

1 whole grain hamburger bun

1 slice Cheddar cheese

½ orange, sliced

Chicken Sausage, Cabbage, and Kidney Bean Sauté

In a medium skillet over medium-high heat, heat 1 teaspoon olive oil. Cook the cabbage, stirring frequently, for 10 minutes, or until soft. Add another teaspoon of olive oil, the chicken sausage, and the beans. Cook, stirring often, for 4 minutes, or until heated through.

Shopping list:

1 cup sliced red cabbage

1 precooked 3-ounce chicken sausage, sliced

1 cup canned kidney beans, rinsed and drained

Per serving: 451 calories, 33 g protein, 50 g carbohydrates, 13 g fiber, 6 g total sugar, 16 g fat, 3 g saturated fat, 526 mg sodium

Chicken Sausage with 'Kraut, Served with Carrot Fries

Preheat the oven to 425°F. Slice the carrots in half widthwise and cut each half into 6 pieces lengthwise to get 24 fry-shaped pieces. Toss with 1 tablespoon olive oil, ⅛ teaspoon salt, and a pinch of cumin and place on a baking sheet. Bake for 20 minutes, turning halfway through, or until golden and crispy on the outside. Meanwhile, in a small skillet over medium-high heat, heat the chicken sausage for 6 minutes, turning several times, or until heated through. Coat the bun with cooking spray; place into the warm skillet to toast. Place the sausage in the bun. Top with 1 teaspoon mustard and the sauerkraut. Serve with the carrot fries and 2 tablespoons ketchup.

Shopping list:

2 large carrots

1 precooked 3-ounce chicken sausage

1 whole grain hot dog bun

⅓ cup sauerkraut

Per serving: 456 calories, 22 g protein, 49 g carbohydrates, 9 g fiber, 20 g total sugar, 22 g fat, 4 g saturated fat, 1,500 mg sodium

The Sugar Smart Express Skinny on Spreadable Fruit and Fruit Juice

Good to know: One teaspoon of 100% spreadable fruit, or ¼ cup of fruit juice, goes a long way toward sweetening up your menu. Here are a few ways to enjoy both.

- Mix spreadable fruit into fat-free plain yogurt, or stir it into plain cooked oats.
- Whisk spreadable fruit into balsamic vinegar and olive oil to make a fruit vinaigrette without a ton of added sugar.

- Use fruit juice to tenderize meat and fish in a marinade, as a base for sauces, or to add brightness to a salad dressing.

Sweet 'n' healthy: Unlike most commercial jams and jellies, 100% fruit spread contains no added sugars. Its sweetness comes from the sugar in the fruit itself. What about fruit juice? With no fiber to slow its journey through your digestive system, it's not a great idea to drink it by the glassful. Use fruit juice as a Flavor Booster, however, and the most you'll use per serving is ¼ cup, which contains around 1 teaspoon of sugar.

Get the best: Treat yourself to a top-of-the-line brand. I like Crofter's Just Fruit Spread Organic Blackberry, which contains 10 calories, 3 grams carbohydrates, and 3 grams sugar per 1 teaspoon. A less expensive alternative, but just as tasty, is Smucker's Simply Fruit Spreadable Fruit: 1 teaspoon contains 13 calories, 3 grams carbohydrates, and 3 grams sugar. How about fruit juice? For orange juice, fresh-squeezed is a good option, since none of the recipes call for more juice than one orange would provide. Otherwise, R. W. Knudsen's Just Juice line is great and contains no added sugar.

Hearty Spinach Salad Vinaigrette with Steak, Strawberries, White Beans, and Pistachios

Whisk together 1 teaspoon olive oil, 2 teaspoons balsamic vinegar, the garlic, and ⅛ teaspoon sea salt; set aside. Toss the spinach with the strawberries, beans, and the dressing. Top with the sliced steak and the pistachios.

Per serving: 450 calories, 32 g protein, 40 g carbohydrates, 10 g fiber, 5 g total sugar, 19 g fat, 5 g saturated fat, 254 mg sodium

Shopping list:

¼ teaspoon minced garlic

1½ cups spinach

3 large strawberries, sliced

⅔ cup canned white beans, rinsed and drained

3 ounces cooked steak

1 tablespoon chopped pistachios

Pepper Stuffed with Turkey, Wild Rice, and Pistachios

Preheat the oven to 375°F. Cook the turkey burger according to package instructions. Crumble and mix it with the onion, rice, ⅛ teaspoon sea salt, and pistachios. Stuff the mixture into the pepper and bake, covered in foil, for 45 minutes, or until the pepper starts to soften. Remove the foil and bake for 15 minutes, or until the top of the pepper starts to brown.

Per serving: 460 calories, 29 g protein, 47 g carbohydrates, 8 g fiber, 9 g total sugar, 18 g fat, 4 g saturated fat, 228 mg sodium

Shopping list:

1 lean 4-ounce turkey burger (such as an Applegate Organic Turkey Burger)

2 tablespoons chopped onion

⅔ cup cooked wild rice

2 tablespoons chopped pistachios

1 yellow bell pepper, cored

Pork Chop with Maple Carrots and Wild Rice Pilaf

Preheat the oven to 425°F. In a bowl, mix the maple syrup, 1 teaspoon of the lemon juice, ½ teaspoon olive oil, ⅛ teaspoon sea salt, and a dash of ground cinnamon. Toss with the carrots. Arrange the carrots on a baking sheet coated with cooking spray. Bake the carrots for 25 minutes, stirring once, or until soft. Meanwhile, sprinkle the pork chop with a pinch of salt and pepper. In an ovenproof skillet over medium-high heat, heat ½ teaspoon canola oil. Cook the chop for 6 minutes, turning once. Transfer the skillet to the oven and bake for 6 minutes, or until a thermometer inserted in the center registers 160°F. Let the chop rest for 5 minutes before serving with the wild rice tossed with the remaining 1 teaspoon lemon juice, cranberries, sunflower seeds, a pinch of sea salt, and ⅛ teaspoon dried thyme. Serve with the glazed carrots.

Per serving: 468 calories, 43 g protein, 43 g carbohydrates, 6 g fiber, 12 g total sugar, 13 g fat, 3 g saturated fat, 389 mg sodium

Shopping list:

1 teaspoon maple syrup
2 teaspoons lemon juice
1 cup sliced carrots
1 small bone-in pork chop
½ cup cooked wild rice
1 teaspoon dried cranberries
1 teaspoon sunflower seeds

Steak with Strawberry Compote, Roasted Potatoes, and Roasted Garlic Broccoli

Preheat the oven to 400°F. In a bowl, mix the strawberries, onion, ½ teaspoon olive oil, and 2 teaspoons balsamic vinegar; set aside. Quarter the potato. Toss it with 1 teaspoon olive oil, ⅛ teaspoon sea salt, and a pinch each of black pepper and smoked paprika. Meanwhile, toss the broccoli with ½ teaspoon olive oil, ⅛ teaspoon sea salt, and the garlic. Bake both the potatoes and broccoli for 30 minutes, turning once, or until soft and golden on the outside. In a small skillet over medium-high heat, heat ½ teaspoon canola oil. Cook the steak for 3 minutes, or until a crust forms. Turn and cook for 3 minutes, or until a thermometer inserted in the center registers 145°F for medium-rare. Let the steak rest on a cutting board for 5 minutes before serving. Top with the strawberry mixture and serve the potatoes and broccoli on the side.

Per serving: 454 calories, 28 g protein, 30 g carbohydrates, 7 g fiber, 7 g total sugar, 26 g fat, 7 g saturated fat, 434 mg sodium

Shopping list:

¼ cup chopped strawberries

1 tablespoon finely chopped onion

1 small yellow potato

1½ cups broccoli florets

¼ teaspoon minced garlic

4 ounces sirloin steak

Veggie Burger Wrap with Hummus and Avocado with Chipotle Kale Chips

Preheat the oven to 350°F. Cook the veggie burger according to package directions. Crumble and set aside. Toss the kale with 1 teaspoon olive oil, ⅛ teaspoon sea salt, and a pinch of chili powder. Bake on a baking sheet for 12 minutes, or until crispy but not browned. Spread the hummus onto the tortilla. Add the crumbled veggie burger and avocado. Roll up the tortilla and serve with the kale chips.

Per serving: 450 calories, 18 g protein, 60 g carbohydrates, 11 g fiber, 2 g total sugar, 14 g fat, 1 g saturated fat, 828 mg sodium

Shopping list:

1 veggie burger (such as Amy's California Veggie Burger)

1½ cups torn kale leaves

1½ tablespoons hummus

1 whole grain tortilla (10" diameter)

⅛ avocado, finely chopped

The Sugar Smart Express Skinny on Maple Syrup

Good to know: By law, pure maple syrup—the kind you buy on weekends in Vermont or New Hampshire—can be made only by the evaporation of pure maple sap and may contain no less than 66 percent sugar by weight. It's pricey, but in the amounts you'll use on this plan, it will last a long time.

As with honey, the flavor of pure maple syrup is affected by a variety of factors. With maple syrup, this includes the genetics of the tree the sap was tapped from, the composition of the soil, weather conditions, and the time during the season when the sap was collected. Besides that can't-be-replicated maple flavor, you might taste hints of caramel, vanilla, nuts, butter, chocolate, or coffee.

Sweet 'n' healthy: While more than 300 different natural compounds are found in pure maple syrup, only one (sugar furanone) is linked to the maple flavor present in all maple syrup. Regardless of flavor, all pure maple syrup is rich in antioxidants. To date, more than 50 have been identified, including polyphenols, which appear to slow enzymes that help convert carbohydrates to sugar. This particular ability raises the possibility of a new way to manage type 2 diabetes.

Get the best: Maple syrup is classified by its color. The darker the syrup, the more intense its flavors. You'll find two types on the market, Grade A and Grade B. Grade A syrup comes in three amber shades: light, medium, and dark. The flavor profile ranges from mild and delicate to strong and caramel-like. Grade B syrup is darker and more maple-y, and it typically costs less than Grade A.

Store it right: Buy your syrup in a glass bottle. Plastic can affect the syrup's color and flavor after 3 to 6 months of storage. Glass, while more expensive, protects the quality of the syrup for a longer period. Unopened, maple syrup will stay fresh for more than a year. After you open it, it will keep in your refrigerator for about 6 months.

Snack Choices (1 per Day—100 Calories)

Basic Fruit and Protein

Serve the egg with the strawberries.

Per serving: 95 calories, 7 g protein, 6 g carbohydrates, 1 g fiber, 4 g total sugar, 5 g fat, 2 g saturated fat, 71 mg sodium

Shopping list:

1 egg, hard cooked

4 large strawberries

Cocoa-Coconut Sliced Banana

Cut the banana into 4 slices width-wise. Dip the top of each slice into unsweetened cocoa powder (1 teaspoon total) and the bottom into the shredded coconut.

Per serving: 85 calories, 1 g protein, 17 g carbohydrates, 3 g fiber, 9 g total sugar, 2 g fat, 2 g saturated fat, 2 mg sodium

Shopping list:

½ banana

2 teaspoons unsweetened shredded coconut

Creamy Avocado-Bean Wedge with Lemon

Spread the avocado wedge with the kidney beans. Drizzle with the lemon juice and a pinch of sea salt.

Per serving: 97 calories, 4 g protein, 11 g carbohydrates, 4 g fiber, <1 g total sugar, 5 g fat, <1 g saturated fat, 59 mg sodium

Shopping list:

¼ avocado

3 tablespoons canned kidney beans, mashed

½ teaspoon lemon juice

Pepper Slices and Chunky Yogurt-Salsa Dip

Add the salsa to the yogurt; stir. Serve as a dip with the bell pepper.

Per serving: 102 calories, 6 g protein, 15 g carbohydrates, 4 g fiber, 12 g total sugar, 2 g fat, <1 g saturated fat, 232 mg sodium

Shopping list:

3 tablespoons chunky salsa

⅓ cup low-fat plain yogurt

1 cup sliced bell pepper

Pistachio-Ginger Kiwi Boats

Cut the kiwifruit in half. Sprinkle each half with ginger and half of the pistachios.

Per serving: 102 calories, 3 g protein, 14 g carbohydrates, 3 g fiber, 8 g total sugar, 5 g fat, <1 g saturated fat, 3 mg sodium

Shopping list:

1 kiwifruit

Pinch grated fresh ginger

4 teaspoons chopped pistachios

Sweet Dreams!

Before Bed, Try This Power-Down Pose

Yoga asanas were designed to calm the body and quiet the mind, preparing the yogi for meditation. The deepest meditative state, called yoga nidra, is known as sleepless sleep—the mind is conscious of its surroundings, but the body is fully relaxed. While I don't expect you to become a yogi, the simple pose below can help you gently shut down your body and mind so that you can slip into sweet, sweet slumber. (You'll want to choose a carpeted area or roll out your yoga mat.)

- Dim the lights and lie on your back.
- Bend your knees, placing your heels close to your butt and hip-width apart.
- Lift your hips off the floor or mat, pushing your pelvis toward the ceiling.
- Arch up onto your shoulders, then lace your fingers together underneath your body as you press your arms into the floor or mat.
- Hold the pose as you take 10 to 15 long, slow breaths.

Snack Choices (1 per Day—150 Calories)

Banana-Strawberry Muesli

Stir the oats and banana into the yogurt. Top with the strawberries, cranberries, and chopped pistachios.

Per serving: 147 calories, 5 g protein, 27 g carbohydrates, 3 g fiber, 14 g total sugar, 3 g fat, <1 g saturated fat, 41 mg sodium

Shopping list:

2 tablespoons rolled oats

¼ very ripe banana, mashed

¼ cup low-fat plain yogurt

2 large strawberries, sliced

1 tablespoon dried cranberries

1 teaspoon chopped pistachios

Creamy-Fruity Ricotta with Honey

Mix the ricotta cheese with the kiwi fruit and strawberries. Drizzle with the honey.

Per serving: 164 calories, 8 g protein, 23 g carbohydrates, 3 g fiber, 15 g total sugar, 5 g fat, 3 g saturated fat, 80 mg sodium

Shopping list:

¼ cup part-skim ricotta cheese

1 kiwifruit, chopped

2 large strawberries, chopped

1 teaspoon honey

Green Tea–Cucumber Smoothie

In a blender, combine the yogurt, green tea, cucumber, banana, and kiwifruit. Blend for 90 seconds, or until smooth. Add 3 ice cubes and blend for 45 seconds, or until all of the ice is smooth.

Per serving: 141 calories, 5 g protein, 30 g carbohydrates, 4 g fiber, 19 g total sugar, 2 g fat, <1 g saturated fat, 44 mg sodium

Shopping list:

¼ cup low-fat plain yogurt

⅓ cup cold unsweetened green tea

¼ cucumber, peeled

½ very ripe banana

1 kiwifruit

South of the Border English Muffin

Toast the English muffin. Top it with the cheese and salsa. Microwave on high power for 25 seconds, or until the cheese is melted.

Per serving: 152 calories, 8 g protein, 14 g carbohydrates, 2 g fiber, 3 g total sugar, 7 g fat, 4 g saturated fat, 313 mg sodium

Shopping list:

½ whole grain English muffin

3 tablespoons shredded Cheddar cheese

1 tablespoon salsa

Strawberry Spice Boats

Slice the strawberries in half lengthwise. Spread each half with ½ teaspoon of the peanut butter and a dash of cinnamon.

Per serving: 147 calories, 6 g protein, 10 g carbohydrates, 3 g fiber, 5 g total sugar, 11 g fat, 2 g saturated fat, 4 mg sodium

Shopping list:

4 large strawberries

4 teaspoons peanut butter

The Sugar Smart Express Skinny on Dried Fruit

Good to know: The intense sweetness of dried fruit is due to the dehydration process. As the water is removed from the fruit, its natural sugars intensify. That shrinkage doesn't just amp up the sweetness. Nutritionists consider dried fruit "energy dense," which means that it packs a ton of calories into a small portion.

Sweet 'n' healthy: The Sugar Smart Express limits the serving size of dried fruit to 2 to 3 tablespoons at a time. That amount yields about 80 calories, around the same number of calories in a piece of whole fruit. But that small amount is plenty sweet as an ingredient in a meal or snack. Your newly sugar-sensitive taste buds will rejoice.

Get the best: Your local supermarket or natural foods store should carry at least a few brands of dried fruits, either packaged or in bulk-bin containers. Wherever you buy, check those ingredients lists for added sugars. Dried cranberries are the one exception to the no-added-sugars rule. Because of their natural tartness, the added sugar brings their sugar level up to that of other dried fruit.

Store it right: Dried fruit doesn't require refrigeration; store it in airtight containers so it doesn't absorb moisture and attract the interest of insects. On occasion, the natural sugars in dried fruit—especially prunes and figs—will solidify, forming crystals on the surface. This is okay. They're still edible, and delicious.

YOU GOT THIS
Managing Stress and Cravings in Phase 3

To help keep you moving along the path to sugar freedom, we're offering some new ways to please your palate, rest up, slow down, and replace emotionally driven urges for sugar with healthy alternatives. Continue to use the Cravings Crushers and the Sweet Freedom strategies from earlier phases, too!

Cravings Crusher: Sip on More "Sweet Waters"

With fresh ingredients like berries and pears, fresh vanilla beans, and zesty ginger, these waters quench your thirst better than sugary drinks do and won't kick up sugar cravings. As you did with the flavored waters in Phase 1 (which you can keep drinking if you like), put the ingredients in a 2-quart jar, muddle with a wooden spoon or spatula, cover with 6 cups of ice, fill the jar with water, and stir. Pop it in the refrigerator for 2 hours to chill and let those luscious flavors mingle. Strain before drinking. Each recipe makes 2 quarts and will keep in the refrigerator for 2 to 3 days.

Berry-Basil Blast

8 fresh basil leaves
3 cups strawberries, halved

Scrunch the basil leaves to release their flavor. Combine with the berries.

Just Peachy

2 vanilla beans
6 peaches, pitted and sliced

Gently crush the beans and stir into the peaches.

Pear-Fect Ginger

10 slices fresh ginger
5 pears, cored and sliced

Stir the ginger and pears together.

Sweet Freedom Strategy: Swap the Treadmill for the Trail

Tried eyes-closed meditation, but can't sit still long enough to reap its benefits? Try a different approach: Take your walk or workout outdoors. Studies show that outdoor exercise confers some of the same benefits as meditation. A review of 11 studies involving 833 people, published in the journal *Environmental Science and Technology,* found that exercising in natural environments was associated with feeling more revitalized and positive, and less stressed, angry, and depressed, compared to exercising indoors. There's even evidence that exercising outside may feel easier (a definite perk!). Whether you're running, walking, or biking outdoors, lift up your eyes and engage your senses, drinking in every sensation—the breeze on your face, the crunch of those leaves, the chirp of birds. That's meditation, too!

I spent *years* traveling in a straight line from home to office and back again at the end of the day. Last year, I decided I absolutely needed to get outside every day—not just to get in my daily walk, but to smell the proverbial roses and feel the sun on my face. I also knew that, however much I desired this, I'd need help making it happen.

Enter CoCo, my beloved, dark-as-bittersweet-chocolate lab. When she was a puppy, I walked her morning, noon, and night. Those half-dozen walks a day gave me plenty of exercise and fresh air.

Although CoCo's since settled down (a lot!), we still take our 15-minute walks each morning, and I treat her (and myself!) to a long hike on the weekend. CoCo is a wonderful antidote to my I'm-too-busy-to-get-outside excuse. The minute we burst out the back door, my stress melts away and her tail starts wagging. Her eagerness to hit the road is contagious—if I had a tail, mine would be wagging, too!

Michelle Davies

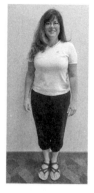

Before starting the Sugar Smart Express, Michelle was pretty much on a sugar high all day long. She'd start her day with a cup of coffee with milk and a heaping teaspoon of sugar. Then she might grab a handful of chocolate chips. Again at lunch, she'd have something sweet to finish her meal. Another cup of sweet coffee, usually with a sugar-laden snack, would get her through the afternoon. And, of course, she'd have dessert after dinner and more coffee. "No meal felt complete to me without something sweet to end it," Michelle says.

And that doesn't count all the hidden sugars and Sugar Mimics Michelle was consuming—carbs like toast with peanut butter and jelly, crackers, and cereal bars.

Michelle's weight got out of control the summer when she and her family moved back to the United States after 8 years in Prague. Suddenly, foods like Doritos and Frosted Mini-Wheats were readily available. "I was eating them all the time as if they were going to go away again," she says. And portion sizes here are enormous. "You don't get endless fries or free drink refills in Europe," says Michelle, who hit her highest weight ever just 2 months after her return. With a family history of obesity, she knew that she had to take control.

Despite going cold turkey on her multiple desserts a day, Michelle continued to bake for her family. To boost her willpower, she focused on a gut feeling she had after starting the program. "I could feel my stomach getting smaller. It felt empty, but not hungry. It wasn't growling. I enjoyed that feeling and didn't want to ruin it by eating dessert," she says.

Since completing the program, Michelle will allow herself a taste of dessert once in a while. But most of the time, she's filling up on avocado slices wrapped in turkey, a Mini Tomato-Chickpea Quesadilla, or Banana-Strawberry Muesli between meals. She's still strict about her coffee, though. Instead of sugar, she adds cinnamon or chia spices. "If I go back to adding sugar, I'll want to eat something sweet with it. And I'm afraid a little would become a heaping teaspoon. This is my line I can't cross."

Seeing the results of all of her hard work makes it worth the effort. Michelle is headache free after years of suffering through three or four a week. And on a recent shopping trip, she was buying size 4s and 6s instead of 8s and 10s. "I haven't been in a size 4 since college."

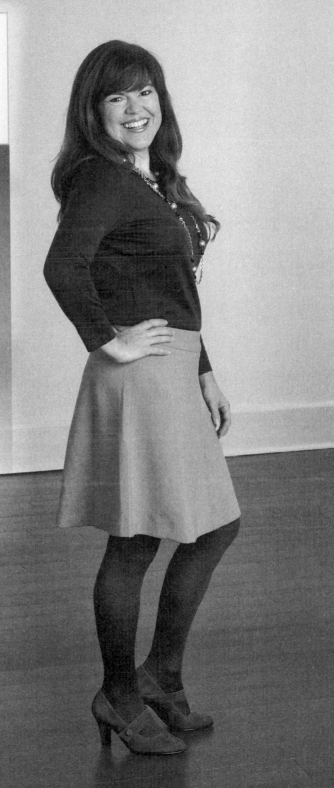

11
POUNDS LOST

AGE:
44

ALL-OVER INCHES LOST:
6.75

SUGAR SMART WISDOM:
"Hang a list of your favorite snacks inside your cabinet. It will serve as a reminder of healthy options the next time you have the munchies."

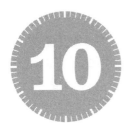

Days 17 to 21: Phase 4

The Sweet Life

PHASE 4 GOALS: To apply your new sugar smarts in the real world, which means staying aware of where added sugar lurks and making informed choices. Also, to realize that you can keep the weight off while savoring the treats you love.

PHASE 4 BENEFITS: By Day 21, you're sure to be feeling as light in spirit as in body. Stress eating is out; mindful eating, daily relaxation time, and sound sleep are in. You're right on the cusp of the sweet life!

Congratulations—you are officially entering the sweet life! At the start of our journey together, I said that sugar isn't evil—that small, sensible amounts won't hurt your health and can soothe your soul. Now it's time to walk that talk. In this final phase, the one you'll follow for life, you're free. Go. Eat a little sugar. Every day, if you want.

My definition of "a little" comes from American Heart Association guidelines: a maximum of 6 teaspoons a day for women, or 9 teaspoons for men. This does *not* include the natural sugar in fruit or other whole foods, just the sugar added to processed foods, or that you stir into or sprinkle onto beverages and foods. For the last 16 days, you've stayed well within these guidelines. In this phase, you'll follow the same eating strategy as in Phase 3, but with one change: You'll add a treat.

The treats in this phase–we're talking Cinnamon-Sugar-Chocolate Toast, Chocolate-Covered Raspberries, and more–contain 100 to 150 calories and a reasonable 3 teaspoons (12 grams) or less of added sugar per serving. Savor one of these sweet delights a day, and you'll still have a few teaspoons of sugar to "spend" any way you like.

I don't know about you, but I'm not spending *any* of my precious teaspoons on ketchup or salad dressing. I choose treats with some nutritional value, like dark chocolate, which contains disease-fighting antioxidants, or whole grain fruit and nut bars, which pack fiber and healthy fats. But that's me. Your 6 teaspoons of sugar are yours. Phase 4 is about knowing your options and feeling free to use them.

For example, in the morning, you might choose to add a teaspoon of sugar (4 grams) to your coffee and a teaspoon of maple syrup (4 grams) to your oatmeal; have a burger on a bun (3 grams) with a tablespoon of ketchup (4 grams) for lunch; do zero sugar grams at dinner; and blow 10 grams on three Twizzlers as your evening snack. That's a total of 25 grams, or just a bit more than 6 teaspoons. Perfect, and satisfying.

In this final phase, as you prepare to rejoin a sugary world, we offer guidance on how to live the sweet life for the rest of your life. Beyond the yummy meals and treats, I've offered you 24 "sugar swaps," which offer name-brand, lower-sugar alternatives to high-sugar products, and advice on what to do if you find your sugar intake creeping up. (For more dining-out advice, see Chapter 11.)

DO THIS
Phase 4 Strategies

- Have breakfast every morning.
- Mix and match the lunch and dinner options. All meals and snacks from Phases 1 through 3 are also allowable. You'll find some new breakfast and lunch/dinner dishes in this phase, as well as some new snacks.
- Enjoy any of the fast-food or chain restaurant meals in Phases 1 through 3.
- Don't forget to snack!
- Optional: Have one serving of a processed grain product per day. In Phase 4, it can be either regular or whole grain. "Once a day" means that if you have a sandwich at lunch, whether on a baguette or on two slices of whole wheat bread, don't have pasta at dinner, even the whole grain variety. As you've learned, Sugar Mimics can negatively affect blood sugar levels. To further reduce the impact of processed grain products, pair them with lean protein, fiber, or a bit of healthy fat.
- Have one serving of fruit up to three times a day.
- Optional: Each day, you may have one meal or snack made with a natural sweetener, such as honey, maple syrup, or dried fruit.
- Treat yourself! In Phase 4 and beyond, you can have a daily serving of sugary food that contains 100 to 150 calories and up to 12 grams of added sugar. (Or not–the treat is optional.) Because of the effect on blood sugar levels, we consider a 6-ounce glass of 100% fruit juice a sugary treat.
- Set your daily intention.

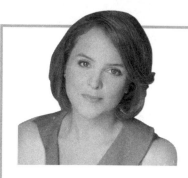

Sweet Inspiration

Ashley Koff, RD

Don't do a "sugar dump." Should you have a latte with sweetened soy milk at the same time as a yogurt with honey or even add fruit to the honey yogurt to make a smoothie, the body is overwhelmed with too much "quick energy." It has to triage, if you will, aiming to send what it can to the cells and set aside (i.e., fat storage) what it doesn't. Not only can the extra sugar lead to weight gain, especially belly fat, but it feeds bad bacteria in your body, negatively impacting the body's immune function and digestive system.

Before caving to a craving, seek its cause. If I notice that my desire for sugar is stronger than usual, I'll first try to identify why. Am I tired, emotional, stressed, dehydrated, or all of the above? To combat any of these, I rely on a magnesium supplement as well as food sources of magnesium (which include the cacao in quality dark chocolate) and look to nonfood fixes (baths, massage, a workout). I also make sure that I am getting enough water and potassium so I stay adequately hydrated.

Give in—with good stuff. When I do get a sugar craving, I will always give into it with a quality source of carbohydrate—like a serving of dark chocolate or organic fruit—so that I don't allow that urge to build into something unmanageable. The human (emotional) brain doesn't like being told that it can't or even that it shouldn't have something. In fact, that can drive an even bigger obsession toward having it.

After a super-sugary treat, monitor your reactions. When I overdo sugar or consume something abnormally sweet (for me)—think birthday cake icing, gelato, candy—there is a tendency for it to stay with me by way of a sugar craving for about 2 more days. So I monitor my consumption more closely on those subsequent days, make sure to get adequate sleep and exercise, and relax to prevent the craving from mounting a stronger offense.

ASHLEY KOFF, RD, maintains an international private practice and is a coauthor of *Mom Energy* and the author of *Recipes for IBS*. She shares her message that better-quality food and supplement choices are the keys to optimal health with millions, regularly appearing on *The Dr. Oz Show*, *The Doctors*, and other TV programs, in magazines (she's *Prevention's* dietitian), on radio, and online at ashleykoffrd.com.

DAILY FOOD LOG

Date:

Today's intention:

Place an X next to the meals and snacks you ate today. You can mix and match your meals and snacks from Phases 1, 2, 3, and 4. Boldface indicates an option added in this phase; an asterisk denotes a recipe that can be found in Chapters 7, 8, or 9.

BREAKFAST

Hunger level _____

__**Bacon 'n' Egg Cup with Avocado Toast**
__Banana-Ricotta Pancakes*
__Basil-Mozzarella Pancakes*
__Breakfast Brown Rice Fritter*
__**Breakfast Pizza**
__Breakfast Tostada*
__Cinnamon-Vanilla Egg White Crepes with Almond Butter Cream*
__Creamy Mocha Frost*
__Deviled Egg Breakfast Sandwich*
__Kiwi-Strawberry Muesli Parfait*
__Loaded Toast*

__Mushroom-Sausage Breakfast Bowl*
__**Orange-Cream Stuffed French Toast**
__**Orange-Raspberry-Almond Smoothie**
__Pumpkin Spice Oats*
__**Raspberry-Ginger-Cashew Oatmeal**
__Starbucks Spinach and Feta Breakfast Wrap*
__Sunny Grape-Buckwheat Breakfast Bowl*
__Sweet Delight Overnight Oat and Chia Pudding*

LUNCH AND DINNER

Hunger level _____

__**BLT Pasta**
__California Roast Beef Pita Sandwich*
__Carrot Slaw with Edamame*
__**Cheddar-Topped Bean, Tomato, and Onion Sauté**
__Cheddar Turkey Burger with Broccoli Slaw*
__Chicken Sausage, Cabbage, and Kidney Bean Sauté*

__Chicken Sausage with 'Kraut, Served with Carrot Fries*
__Chipotle Burrito Bowl*
__**Classic Roast Beef Sandwich**
__Creamy-Crispy Tofu Salad*
__Curried Black Bean and Corn Burger over Quinoa Salad*
__**Fennel, Farro, and Chicken Salad**

(continued)

DAILY FOOD LOG (cont.)

__Feta-Mushroom Crab Cake over Basil-Olive Buckwheat*

__Frozen Meal: Artisan Bistro Grass-Fed Beef with Mushroom Sauce*

__**Grilled Chicken, Orange, and Goat Cheese Pita**

__Grilled Chicken and Sweet Potato Sandwich*

__Hearty Spinach Salad Vinaigrette with Steak, Strawberries, White Beans, and Pistachios*

__**Lean Beef Burger with Roasted Fennel and Wild Rice**

__Lemon-Salmon Tabbouleh*

__Outback Steakhouse 6-Ounce Victoria's Filet, Grilled Asparagus, and Baked Potato*

__Oven-"Fried" Tofu Sticks with Creamy Peanut-Soy Dip*

__Panera Bread Chicken Cobb with Avocado*

__Pepper Stuffed with Turkey, Wild Rice, and Pistachios*

__Pork Chop with Maple Carrots and Wild Rice Pilaf*

__Quinoa Enchiladas*

__Rosemary Pork Tenderloin with Parmesan Potato Spears*

__Southwestern Salad with Cilantro Dressing*

__Spiced Turkey-Veggie-Quinoa Scramble/Wrap*

__Starbucks Hearty Veggie and Brown Rice Salad Bowl*

__Steak with Strawberry Compote, Roasted Potatoes, and Roasted Garlic Broccoli*

__Sweet and Savory Brown Rice Salad with Chicken, Cheese, and Greens*

__**Sweet 'n' Savory Waffles**

__**Tomato-and-Veggie Eggs with Pita**

__Tomato, Onion, and Parmesan Salmon Frittata*

__**Tortilla Pizza with Egg, Veggies, and Mozzarella**

__Tuna Niçoise Salad*

__Tuna Tacos with Zucchini Slaw, Spicy Yogurt Sauce, and Salsa Brown Rice*

__Turkey Sausage–Mushroom-Onion Stuffed Baked Potato with Roasted Cauliflower*

__Veggie Burger Wrap with Hummus and Avocado with Chipotle Kale Chips*

__Whole Grain Penne with Ricotta, Grape Tomatoes, and Broccoli*

__**Wild Rice, Broccolini, and White Bean Bowl with Cashews**

SNACKS (100 CALORIES)

Hunger level _____

__Asian Edamame and Carrot Salad*

__Basic Fruit and Protein*

__**Chocolate-Covered Raspberries**

__Chopped Apple, Feta, and Mint Salad*

__Cocoa-Coconut Sliced Banana*

__Creamy Avocado-Bean Wedge with Lemon*

__Cumin–Black Bean Dip with Carrots*

__**Fennel with White Bean Dip**

__Frozen Banana–Almond Butter Sandwiches*

__**Homemade Chocolate Milk**

__**Mini Omelet**

__Mini Tomato-Chickpea Quesadilla*

__Orange with **Cashew-Honey-Yogurt Dip**

__Pepper Slices and Chunky Yogurt-Salsa Dip*

__Pistachio-Ginger Kiwi Boats*

__**Roast Beef Wrap with Tomato and Avocado**

__Salmon and Corn Salad*

__Tomato-Parmesan Bites*

__Tuna and Chopped Olives with Lemon and Dried Dillweed*

__**Zucchini Boats Stuffed with Goat Cheese and Chives**

SNACKS (150 CALORIES)

Hunger level _____

__Apple Slices with Chia-Yogurt Drizzle*

__Banana-Strawberry Muesli*

__Cauliflower Florets and Hummus*

__Chili-Spiced Turkey Avocado Roll-Ups*

__**Cinnamon-Sugar-Chocolate Toast**

__Cinnamon-Walnut Quinoa*

__Creamy-Fruity Ricotta with Honey*

__Creamy Kale Salad*

__Crisp-Roasted Cinnamon Chickpeas*

__Green Tea–Cucumber Smoothie*

__**Microwave S'more**

Orange-Spice Vanilla Pudding

__South of the Border English Muffin*

__Strawberry Ba-Nilla Snack Smoothie*

__**Strawberry No-Bake Cheesecake Parfait**

__Strawberry Spice Boats*

__Whole Grain Crispbread with Almond Butter and Sliced Grapes*

ADDITIONAL FOODS

NOTES

SHOP THIS

Choose your meals and customize your shopping list. Each recipe is a single serving. If you're cooking for two or more people, multiply the ingredient quantities by the number of servings you want to make.

EAT THIS
Phase 4 Quick & Easy Meals

Have three meals and two snacks every day from the options below.

Breakfast Choices

Bacon 'n' Egg Cup with Avocado Toast

Preheat the oven to 350°F. In a small skillet over medium-high heat, cook the bacon until lightly browned but still flexible. Set aside. Coat 1 cup of a muffin tin with cooking spray and wrap the bacon around the inside of the cup. Crack the egg into the center of the cup; add the egg white. Bake for 15 minutes, or until the egg white is set and the yolk is firm. Serve with the crispbread spread with the avocado and sprinkled with paprika.

Shopping list:
1 slice center-cut bacon
1 egg + 1 egg white
1 whole grain crispbread
¼ avocado, mashed

Per serving: 307 calories, 15 g protein, 24 g carbohydrates, 6 g fiber, 4 g total sugar, 17 g fat, 4 g saturated fat, 509 mg sodium

---

The Strawberry No-Bake Cheesecake Parfait—simple and delicious! —Linda

---

Breakfast Pizza

Preheat the broiler. Top each half of
the English muffin with half of the
tomatoes, spinach, turkey sausage,
and mozzarella cheese. Broil for
3 minutes, or until the cheese is
melted and golden.

Per serving: 292 calories, 19 g protein, 33 g carbohydrates,
5 g fiber, 6 g total sugar, 10 g fat, 5 g saturated fat,
645 mg sodium

Shopping list:

1 whole grain English muffin

2 tablespoons canned chopped
tomatoes

2 tablespoons chopped spinach

¼ cup cooked crumbled turkey
sausage

¼ cup shredded part-skim
mozzarella cheese

Orange-Cream Stuffed French Toast

Spread the cream cheese onto the
bread. Slice the bread on the
diagonal. Chop the orange; mix in
the honey. Center the honey-orange
mixture on 1 diagonal slice. Top with
the other slice, cream cheese side
down, to form a sandwich. Press the
edges slightly to seal in the orange
mixture. Whisk the egg and egg white
with ½ teaspoon vanilla extract and
the milk. Dip the stuffed bread into
the egg mixture, allowing it to soak
for 3 to 4 minutes. Fry in ½ teaspoon
canola oil over medium-high heat for
6 minutes, turning once, or until firm
and golden.

Per serving: 316 calories, 15 g protein, 37 g carbohydrates,
6 g fiber, 16 g total sugar, 13 g fat, 5 g saturated fat,
327 mg sodium

Shopping list:

2 tablespoons reduced-fat
cream cheese

1 slice whole grain bread

½ orange, peeled

1 teaspoon honey

1 egg + 1 egg white

1 tablespoon fat-free milk

Orange-Raspberry-Almond Smoothie

In a blender, combine the orange, raspberries, carrot, milk, and almond butter. Blend on high for 1 minute, or until smooth. Add 4 ice cubes and blend on high for 45 seconds, or until all of the ice is smooth.

Per serving: 308 calories, 15 g protein, 45 g carbohydrates, 11 g fiber, 31 g total sugar, 10 g fat, 1 g saturated fat, 180 mg sodium

Shopping list:
1 orange, peeled
½ cup raspberries
1 carrot, chopped
1 cup fat-free milk
1 tablespoon almond butter

Raspberry-Ginger-Cashew Oatmeal

In a small food processor or blender, combine ⅓ cup raspberries and the strawberry fruit spread. Process or blend until pureed, adding 1 teaspoon water if needed. Whisk the oats, milk, raspberry puree, and ⅛ teaspoon ground ginger (or ½ teaspoon fresh grated) in a small saucepan over high heat. Once the mixture comes to a boil, reduce the heat to medium-low and simmer for 10 minutes, or until the oats are soft and thick. Top with ¼ cup raspberries and the cashews.

Per serving: 310 calories, 13 g protein, 44 g carbohydrates, 9 g fiber, 13 g total sugar, 15 g fat, 2 g saturated fat, 92 mg sodium

Shopping list:
⅓ cup + ¼ cup raspberries
1 teaspoon 100% fruit strawberry fruit spread
⅓ cup rolled oats
⅔ cup fat-free milk
2 tablespoons chopped toasted cashews

Lunch and Dinner Choices

BLT Pasta

In a small food processor or blender, combine the white beans with the lemon juice, ¼ teaspoon sea salt, garlic, a pinch of black pepper, and 1 tablespoon warm water. Process or blend until smooth. Set aside. In a small skillet over medium-high heat, cook the bacon for 4 minutes, or until just crispy. Remove the bacon from the pan, crumble, and set aside. In the same pan, cook the lettuce with a pinch of pepper for 2 minutes, stirring frequently, or until just wilted. Toss the penne with the white bean puree and gently mix with the bacon and lettuce and tomatoes.

Per serving: 448 calories, 26 g protein, 65 g carbohydrates, 11 g fiber, 4 g total sugar, 11 g fat, 4 g saturated fat, 1,174 mg sodium

Shopping list:

- ½ cup canned white beans, rinsed and drained
- 1 tablespoon lemon juice
- ½ clove garlic
- 2 slices center-cut bacon
- 1 cup chopped romaine lettuce (no outer leaves)
- 1 cup cooked whole grain penne
- ¼ cup halved grape tomatoes

Cheddar-Topped Bean, Tomato, and Onion Sauté

In a medium skillet over medium-high heat, heat 1 teaspoon olive oil. Cook the onion and tomatoes for 8 minutes, or until the onion is golden and the tomatoes have wrinkled. Add the beans and 1 teaspoon olive oil; cook for 3 minutes, or until steaming hot. Remove from the heat and sprinkle with the cheese. Let sit for 2 minutes to melt the cheese.

Per serving: 456 calories, 22 g protein, 45 g carbohydrates, 2 g fiber, 6 g total sugar, 22 g fat, 8 g saturated fat, 578 mg sodium

Shopping list:
¼ cup chopped onion
1 cup grape tomatoes
1 cup canned pinto beans, rinsed and drained
⅓ cup shredded Cheddar cheese

Classic Roast Beef Sandwich

Spread the mayonnaise onto 1 slice of the bread. Top with the roast beef, 2 slices tomato, lettuce, and other slice of bread.

Per serving: 446 calories, 23 g protein, 43 g carbohydrates, 9 g fiber, 8 g total sugar, 19 g fat, 4 g saturated fat, 413 mg sodium

Shopping list:
1 tablespoon mayonnaise
2 slices whole grain bread
3 slices lean deli roast beef
2 slices tomato
1 large leaf romaine lettuce

Fennel, Farro, and Chicken Salad

In a bowl, toss the fennel with the chicken breast, apricots, and farro. In another bowl, whisk the lemon juice, 1 tablespoon olive oil, ⅛ teaspoon sea salt, and a pinch each of garlic powder, chili powder, cumin, and smoked paprika. Add the dressing to the fennel mixture; toss to coat.

Per serving: 465 calories, 33 g protein, 44 g carbohydrates, 7 g fiber, 3 g total sugar, 18 g fat, 3 g saturated fat, 303 mg sodium

Shopping list:
½ small bulb fennel, thinly sliced
½ cup chopped cooked skinless chicken breast
2 teaspoons chopped dried apricots
¾ cup cooked farro
1 tablespoon lemon juice

Grilled Chicken, Orange, and Goat Cheese Pita

Whisk together 1 teaspoon olive oil, the lemon juice, strawberry fruit spread, ⅛ teaspoon sea salt, a pinch of black pepper, and the mint. Set aside. Toss the chicken breast with the orange, goat cheese, and the mint dressing. Stuff into the pita.

Per serving: 473 calories, 35 g protein, 54 g carbohydrates, 7 g fiber, 6 g total sugar, 14 g fat, 5 g saturated fat, 717 mg sodium

Shopping list:
1 teaspoon lemon juice
½ teaspoon 100% fruit strawberry fruit spread
1 teaspoon chopped fresh mint
½ cup chopped grilled skinless chicken breast
⅓ orange, peeled and chopped
2 tablespoons crumbled goat cheese
1 whole grain pita (6" diameter)

Lean Beef Burger with Roasted Fennel and Wild Rice

Preheat the oven to 425°F. Toss the with 1 teaspoon olive oil and ⅛ teaspoon sea salt. Place on a baking sheet and bake for 25 minutes, turning once, or until soft and just starting to turn golden. Mix the onion, bell pepper, ¼ teaspoon of the garlic, and a pinch of black pepper with the ground beef. In a skillet over medium-high heat, heat 1 teaspoon canola oil. Cook the burger for 10 minutes, turning once, or until a thermometer inserted in the center registers 160°F and the meat is no longer pink. Serve the burger over the wild rice tossed with the cashews, the remaining ¼ teaspoon garlic, and ⅛ teaspoon salt, with the fennel on the side.

Per serving: 443 calories, 15 g protein, 56 g carbohydrates, 6 g fiber, 4 g total sugar, 18 g fat, 3 g saturated fat, 398 mg sodium

Shopping list:

- ½ bulb fennel, thinly sliced
- 2 tablespoons chopped onion
- 1 tablespoon chopped bell pepper
- ½ teaspoon minced garlic
- 4 ounces lean ground beef
- 1 cup wild rice, cooked
- 1 tablespoon chopped roasted cashews

Sweet 'n' Savory Waffle

Preheat the oven to 400°F. In a bowl, toss the carrots with ½ teaspoon olive oil and the orange juice. Spread on a baking sheet and roast for 15 minutes. Meanwhile, in a skillet, cook the egg in ½ teaspoon olive oil to desired doneness. Top the waffles with the turkey sausage, egg, and maple syrup. Serve with the carrots on the side.

Per serving: 476 calories, 20 g protein, 53 g carbohydrates, 6 g fiber, 22 g total sugar, 22 g fat, 6 g saturated fat, 743 mg sodium

Shopping list:
1 cup sliced carrots
1 tablespoon orange juice
1 egg
2 whole grain frozen waffles
¼ cup cooked crumbled turkey breakfast sausage
2 teaspoons maple syrup

Tomato-and-Veggie Eggs with Pita

In a small skillet with a lid over medium-high heat, heat 1 teaspoon olive oil. Add the onion, pepper, zucchini, ⅛ teaspoon smoked paprika, and ⅛ teaspoon salt. Cook, stirring frequently, for 12 minutes, or until the veggies are soft. Add the beans and tomatoes. Heat until lightly bubbling. Make 2 wells in the center of the pan; add a raw egg to each well. Cook for 3 minutes, or until the egg whites begin to turn white. Place a lid on the pan and cook for 3 minutes, or until the eggs are just cooked through. Sprinkle with the parsley and serve with the pita.

Per serving: 465 calories, 24 g protein, 57 g carbohydrates, 9 g fiber, 13 g total sugar, 16 g fat, 4 g saturated fat, 1,073 mg sodium

Shopping list:
⅓ cup chopped yellow onion
⅓ cup chopped bell pepper
⅓ cup chopped zucchini
⅓ cup canned pinto beans, rinsed and drained
1 cup canned chopped tomatoes
2 eggs
1 teaspoon chopped fresh parsley
½ whole wheat pita (6"diameter)

Tortilla Pizza with Egg, Veggies, and Mozzarella

Preheat the broiler. In a skillet, cook the egg with ½ teaspoon olive oil to desired doneness. Coat 1 side of the tortilla with cooking spray. Broil for 2 minutes, turning once, or until the edges begin to crisp. Spread the tomatoes over the tortilla. Add the onion, bell pepper, and mozzarella cheese. Place under the broiler for 2 minutes, or until the cheese is melted and golden. Top with the egg.

Per serving: 437 calories, 24 g protein, 51 g carbohydrates, 8 g fiber, 6 g total sugar, 16 g fat, 7 g saturated fat, 830 mg sodium

Shopping list:

1 egg

1 whole grain tortilla (10″ diameter)

½ cup canned chopped tomatoes

2 tablespoons chopped onion

¼ cup chopped bell pepper

⅓ cup shredded part-skim mozzarella cheese

Wild Rice, Broccolini, and White Bean Bowl with Cashews

In a small skillet over medium-high heat, heat 1 teaspoon olive oil. Cook the Broccolini for 5 minutes, stirring frequently, or until soft and wilted. Toss with 1 teaspoon of the soy sauce and 1 teaspoon of the lemon juice. Mix the rice with the beans, remaining 1 teaspoon soy sauce, remaining 1 teaspoon lemon juice, and the garlic. Top the rice mixture with the Broccolini and cashews.

Per serving: 442 calories, 20 g protein, 71 g carbohydrates, 13 g fiber, 2 g total sugar, 10 g fat, 2 g saturated fat, 383 mg sodium

Shopping list:

1½ cups Broccolini

2 teaspoons reduced-sodium soy sauce

2 teaspoons lemon juice

⅔ cup cooked wild rice

¾ cup canned white beans, rinsed and drained

¼ teaspoon minced garlic

1 tablespoon chopped roasted cashews

Snack Choices (1 per Day—100 Calories)

Chocolate-Covered Raspberries

In a microwaveable bowl, mix the chocolate chips with the milk. Microwave on medium power for 10 seconds. Stir and microwave for 10 more seconds. Stir again. Repeat in 10 second-increments until the mixture is smooth. Arrange the raspberries on a parchment-lined baking sheet. Drizzle the chocolate over the berries. Place the baking sheet in the freezer for 10 minutes to set.

Per serving: 100 calories, 2 g protein, 16 g carbohydrates, 5 g fiber, 11 g total sugar, 4 g fat, 2 g saturated fat, 7 mg sodium

Shopping list:
1½ tablespoons dark chocolate chips
2 teaspoons fat-free milk
½ cup fresh raspberries

Fennel with White Bean Dip

In a blender, combine the beans, lemon juice, ½ teaspoon olive oil, ⅛ teaspoon sea salt, 2 teaspoons warm water, and a pinch of black pepper. Blend until smooth. Use as a dip for the fennel.

Per serving: 96 calories, 5 g protein, 14 g carbohydrates, 4 g fiber, 2 g total sugar, 2 g fat, >1 g saturated fat, 205 mg sodium

Shopping list:
¼ cup canned white beans, rinsed and drained
2 teaspoons lemon juice
½ cup sliced fennel

Homemade Chocolate Milk

Whisk together the cocoa powder, maple syrup, and milk or soy milk until smooth. Add 3 to 4 ice cubes to chill.

Per serving: 105 calories, 7 g protein, 20 g carbohydrates, 1 g fiber, 19 g total sugar, <1 g fat, <1 g saturated fat, 80 mg sodium

Shopping list:

2 teaspoons unsweetened cocoa powder

2 teaspoons maple syrup

¾ cup fat-free milk or unsweetened soy milk

Crave Chocolate? Come to the Dark Side

With its distinctive bittersweet taste and "top notes" of coffee, nuts, or cinnamon, dark chocolate is the definitive better-for-you treat. Swap it for milk chocolate, and you'll consume significantly less sugar. But that's not the only reason we swoon for it: Although its flavor isn't traditionally sweet, its health benefits are.

Dark chocolate is rich in antioxidants called flavonoids, which give it its unique "bite" and are responsible for many of its health benefits. For example, flavonoids appear to benefit cardiovascular health by lowering blood pressure, improving bloodflow to the brain and heart, and making blood less sticky, which reduces the risk of heart attack and stroke.

Moreover, compared to milk chocolate, dark chocolate promotes that I'm-full feeling known as satiety, lowers the desire to eat sweets, and reduces calorie intake, which may help with weight loss, a study published in *Nutrition & Diabetes* found. When researchers gave 16 participants 3½ ounces of either dark or milk chocolate and 2 hours later offered them pizza, those who consumed the dark chocolate ate 15 percent fewer calories from the pizza than those who had milk chocolate.

If you're used to milk chocolate, go dark gradually so you train your taste buds to appreciate the stronger taste. Look for a variety that has a 70 percent or higher cacao, or cocoa, content and lists cacao as its first ingredient.

Mini Omelet

Whisk the egg whites with the onion, Cheddar cheese, rice, and a pinch each of sea salt, black pepper, and dried oregano. In a medium skillet over medium-high heat, heat ½ teaspoon olive oil. Cook the egg mixture for 4 minutes, turning once, or until cooked through.

Per serving: 108 calories, 10 g protein, 7 g carbohydrates, >1 g fiber, >1 g total sugar, 5 g fat, 2 g saturated fat, 208 mg sodium

Shopping list:

2 egg whites

2 teaspoons chopped onion

1 tablespoon shredded Cheddar cheese

2 tablespoons cooked wild rice

Orange with Cashew-Honey-Yogurt Dip

Peel the orange half. Divide it into segments. Blend the cashews with the honey and yogurt. Use as a dip.

Per serving: 117 calories, 4 g protein, 10 g carbohydrates, 2 g fiber, 12 g total sugar, 5 g fat, 1 g saturated fat, 30 mg sodium

Shopping list:

½ orange

1 tablespoon chopped roasted cashews

½ teaspoon honey

3 tablespoons low-fat plain yogurt

Roast Beef Wrap with Tomato and Avocado

Lay the tomato on the roast beef. Top with the avocado. Roll up.

Per serving: 107 calories, 9 g protein, 4 g carbohydrates, 3 g fiber, 1 g total sugar, 7 g fat, 1 g saturated fat, 44 mg sodium

Shopping list:
¼ cup chopped tomato
1 slice lean deli roast beef
¼ avocado

Zucchini Boats Stuffed with Goat Cheese and Chives

Cut the zucchini in half lengthwise. Spread each piece with half of the goat cheese and half of the chives.

Per serving: 108 calories, 7 g protein, 4 g carbohydrates, >1 g fiber, 3 g total sugar, 8 g fat, 5 g saturated fat, 111 mg sodium

Shopping list:
½ zucchini
3 tablespoons goat cheese
2 teaspoons chopped chives

FAQs for Phase 4

Q: I love my energy bars, but they tend to contain a lot of sugar, either from fruit or added sugars. Is it okay to have one as a snack?

A: Yes! There are plenty of healthy options to choose from. I'd recommend choosing a bar that contains 200 calories or fewer and at least 3 grams of fiber. Either swap the bar for your treat for the day, or have it for one of your snacks and skip the other snack.

Ingredients like fruit and added sugars matter, too. Here are some guidelines.

- A bar *with* added sugar but *no* fruit: 9 g sugar or less
- A bar with both added sugar and fruit: up to 12 g sugar
- A bar *with* fruit but *no* added sugar: up to 12 g sugar

The fruit is usually a puree of dried fruit, which on this plan counts as added sugar. But dried fruit does contain nutrients, and often these bars provide fiber, healthy fat, and protein in the form of nuts, which slow the breakdown of the sugar in your body. Here are some better-for-you choices.

- Clif Mojo Peanut Butter Pretzel (1 bar), 190 calories, 9 g sugar, 2 g fiber
- Kind Dark Chocolate Nuts and Sea Salt (1 bar), 200 calories, 5 g sugar, 7 g fiber
- Kind Madagascar Vanilla Almond (1 bar), 210 calories, 4 g sugar, 5 g fiber
- Lärabar Über Sticky Bun Sweet and Salty Fruit and Nut Bar (1 bar), 220 calories, 7 g sugar, 3 g fiber

- Luna Blueberry Bliss (1 bar), 180 calories, 13 g sugar, 3 g fiber
- Nature's Path Macaroon Crunch (2 bars), 200 calories, 8 g sugar, 3 g fiber
- Nature's Path Trail Mixer Chewy Granola Bar (1 bar), 140 calories, 9 g sugar, 3 g fiber

Snack Choices (1 per Day—150 Calories)

Cinnamon-Sugar-Chocolate Toast

Mix the sugar, ¼ teaspoon unsweetened cocoa powder, and ⅛ teaspoon ground cinnamon into the butter. Spread on the toast.

Per serving: 151 calories, >1 g protein, 25 g carbohydrates, 4 g fiber, 7 g total sugar, 5 g fat, 3 g saturated fat, 106 mg sodium

Shopping list:

1 teaspoon sugar

1 teaspoon unsalted butter

1 slice whole grain bread, toasted

Microwave S'more

Top ½ graham cracker sheet with the chocolate chips and marshmallows. Microwave on high power for 15 seconds. Continue to microwave in 5-second increments until the chips are soft. Top with the remaining ½ graham cracker.

Per serving: 139 calories, 2 g protein, 27 g carbohydrates, >1 g fiber, 17 g total sugar, 4 g fat, 1 g saturated fat, 97 mg sodium

Shopping list:

1 graham cracker

15 dark chocolate chips

2 regular-size marshmallows

Orange-Spice Vanilla Pudding

Stir a pinch of ground nutmeg into the pudding. Top with the orange and the cashews.

Per serving: 158 calories, 4 g protein, 30 g carbohydrates, 1 g fiber, 22 g total sugar, 3 g fat, >1 g saturated fat, 243 mg sodium

Shopping list:

4 ounces low-fat vanilla pudding (such as Jell-O Vanilla Pudding Cup)

¼ cup chopped orange segments

2 teaspoons chopped roasted cashews

Strawberry No-Bake Cheesecake Parfait

Using a fork, mix the honey and ¼ teaspoon vanilla extract into the cream cheese. Place half of the cream cheese mixture in the bottom of a shot glass. Top with half the crumbled vanilla wafer and 1 large chopped strawberry. Repeat layers.

Shopping list:

2 teaspoons honey

2 tablespoons reduced-fat cream cheese

1 vanilla wafer, crumbled

2 large strawberries, chopped

Per serving: 151 calories, 4 g protein, 21 g carbohydrates, >1 g fiber, 13 g total sugar, 7 g fat, 4 g saturated fat, 108 mg sodium

Sweet Dreams!
Sleep Pink

You've likely heard of white noise, produced when the sounds of different frequencies are combined. It is often touted as a way to ease yourself into sleep. A study published in the *Journal of Theoretical Biology*, however, found that a noise with a prettier name—pink noise—ushered in sleep even better.

Pink noise is a type of sound in which every octave carries the same power, or a perfectly consistent frequency. Think of rain falling on pavement or wind rustling the leaves on a tree. It's called pink noise because light with a similar power spectrum would appear pink.

In the study, conducted to discover how pink noise would affect sleepers, researchers from China exposed 50 volunteers to either no noise or the pink variety during nighttime sleep and daytime naps while monitoring their brain activity. A whopping 75 percent of the participants reported that they slept more restfully when the pink noise was on. When it came to brain activity, the amount of "stable sleep"—the most restful kind—increased 23 percent among the nighttime sleepers exposed to pink noise and more than 45 percent among nappers.

Sound plays a big role in brain activity and brain wave synchronization even while you're sleeping, the study notes. The steady drone of pink noise slows and regulates your brain waves—a hallmark of restful sleep. To try pink sleep for yourself, set up a fan that produces a steady, uninterrupted sound, or use the rain forest setting on a noise machine.

SUGAR SMART SWAPS

Now that you've determined the sugary indulgences you can't live without, it's time to eliminate items that waste precious teaspoons of sugar and identify alternatives that you enjoy just as much. This list of swaps and tips can help.

We've presented our swaps by category, so you can zip down the list and find the items most important to you. You'll find sugar swaps for beverages on page 212. Prepare to discover new, better-for-you indulgences!

Grain Products

Sugar has no place in the bread aisle, but you'd never know it by how many grain products contain added grams.

Swap This . . .	For This . . .
Arnold 100% Whole Wheat Bread (1 slice): 110 calories, 4 g sugar	Food for Life Ezekiel 4:9 Flax Sprouted Whole Grain Bread (1 slice): 80 calories, 0 g sugar
Quaker Instant Oatmeal Maple and Brown Sugar (1 packet): 160 calories, 12 g sugar	Trader Joe's Gluten-Free Rolled Oats (½ cup uncooked): 150 calories, 1 g sugar
Kellogg's Raisin Bran Crunch cereal (1 cup): 190 calories, 19 g sugar	Post Shredded Wheat cereal (1 cup): 170 calories, 0 g sugar
Bisquick Complete Pancake and Waffle Mix Simply Buttermilk with Whole Grain (½ cup): 210 calories, 6 g sugar	Bob's Red Mill Organic 7 Grain Pancake and Waffle Whole Grain Mix (⅓ cup): 190 calories, 2 g sugar

Condiments, Sauces, and Dressings

When it comes to your sugar allowance, waste not. Balsamic vinegar, pure olive oil, herbs, spices, hot sauce, salsa, and natural sweeteners add plenty of flavor without added sugars.

Swap This . . .	For This . . .
Newman's Own Creamy Balsamic dressing (1 tablespoon): 50 calories, 4 g sugar	Newman's Own Creamy Caesar dressing (1 tablespoon): 85 calories, 0 g sugar
Bertolli Tomato & Basil Sauce (½ cup): 70 calories, 12 g sugar	Monte Bene Tomato Basil Pasta Sauce (½ cup): 40 calories, <1 g sugar
Smucker's Strawberry Jam (1 tablespoon): 50 calories, 12 g sugar	Polaner All Fruit Strawberry (1 tablespoon): 35 calories, 7 g sugar
La Choy Stir Fry Orange Ginger Sauce and Marinade (1 tablespoon): 25 calories, 4 g sugar	La Choy Stir Fry Teriyaki Sauce and Marinade (1 tablespoon): 10 calories, 1 g sugar

Sweet Treats

Skeptical? Just give them a try. One taste of the low-sugar indulgences on this list (we've sampled them all) and you'll never miss the sugar-laden items.

Swap This . . .	For This . . .
Twix (1 package): 250 calories, 24 g sugar	Dagoba Organic Chocolate Xocolatl dark chocolate bar 74% cacao (1 ounce): 140 calories, 7 g sugar
Entenmann's Deluxe French Cheesecake (1 serving): 390 calories, 25 g sugar	Yasso Frozen Greek Yogurt bars (1 coconut bar): 80 calories, 12 g sugar
Premium ice cream, vanilla (½ cup): 266 calories, 22 g sugar	Creamies Reduced Fat Ice Cream Bar (1 strawberry bar): 120 calories, 13 g sugar
Oreos (3): 160 calories, 14 g sugar	Walkers Shortbread fingers (2 cookies): 150 calories, 4 g sugar
Gummy worms (10 worms): 293 calories, 44 g sugar	Tasty Brand Organic Wild Berry Fruit Snacks (1 pouch, 23 g): 70 calories, 10 g sugar

Peanut Butter, Yogurt, and Miscellaneous

You won't miss the sugar in these swaps–the natural sugars in peanuts, yogurt, and fruit products are sweet enough on their own!

Swap This . . .	For This . . .
Jif Peanut Butter (2 tablespoons): 190 calories, 3 g sugar	Smucker's Organic Peanut Butter (2 tablespoons): 210 calories, 1 g sugar
Stonyfield Organic Fat-Free French Vanilla Yogurt (8 ounces): 170 calories, 33 g sugar	Siggi's Icelandic Style Skyr Strained Nonfat Yogurt, Pomegranate & Passion Fruit (5.3 ounces): 100 calories, 9 g sugar
Healthy Choice Modern Classics Sweet and Sour Chicken: 390 calories, 19 g sugar	Weight Watchers Smart Ones Bistro Selections Slow Roasted Turkey Breast: 200 calories, 1 g sugar
Mott's Original Applesauce (sweetened, 4 ounces): 90 calories, 22 g sugar	Mott's Natural Applesauce (unsweetened, 4 ounces): 50 calories, 11 g sugar
Del Monte Peach Chunks in Heavy Syrup (½ cup): 100 calories, 21 g sugar	Dole Frozen Sliced Peaches (¾ cup): 50 calories, 10 g sugar

Liquid Treats

Sweetened beverages such as sodas, sweetened teas and waters, and specialty coffee drinks count toward your daily added-sugar allotment. We count 100% fruit juice as an added sugar because juice has no fiber to slow the digestion of the sugar. While none of our swaps includes artificial sweeteners, we recommend all-natural thirst quenchers like water, seltzer, green tea, black tea, and coffee. (You can put milk or cream and a teaspoon of honey or sugar in your coffee or tea, if you want.) If you haven't yet mixed up a pitcher of one of our flavored waters (Chapters 7 and 9) or tried our DIY flavored coffee (on the opposite page), give them a try.

Swap This . . .	For This . . .
Sprite (12 ounces): 140 calories, 38 g sugar	8 ounces seltzer mixed with 4 ounces 100% fruit juice: 55 calories, 11 g sugar (if made with orange juice)

Swap This . . .	For This . . .
Starbucks Hot Chocolate, made with fat-free milk and no whipped cream (8 ounces): 130 calories, 23 g sugar	Homemade Chocolate Milk (page 204), served warm (8 ounces): 105 calories, 19 g sugar
Snapple Green Tea (16 ounces): 120 calories, 30 g sugar	Honest Tea Organic Assam Black Tea (16 ounces): 35 calories, 9 g sugar
Welch's Grape Juice (8 ounces): 140 calories, 36 g sugar	R.W. Knudsen Family Just Cranberry juice (8 ounces): 70 calories, 9 g sugar
Arizona Rx Energy Herbal Tonic (23 ounces): 345 calories, 83 g sugar	Sweet Leaf Unsweet Tea, Lemon and Lime (16 ounces): 0 calories, 0 g sugar

YOU GOT THIS
Managing Stress and Cravings in Phase 4

With 3 weeks of healthy, low-sugar eating under your belt, which I'm betting you've taken in a notch or two, you're ready to apply your sugar smarts. I send you off with one last round of tips for outwitting sugar cravings and stress eating. Give them a try, and keep using those you learned in previous phases.

Cravings Crusher: Swap a Sugary Coffee Drink for This

Specialty coffee shop drinks—like sugar-packed Frappuccinos and syrup-laced options—help grow sugar bellies, even if you don't add a scone to your coffee order. If you're hooked on coffee drinks, try our no-sugar, low-cal indulgence. At just 100 calories a serving, with zero sugar, it tastes decadent. (We used mocha-flavored coffee, but it tastes just as good made with vanilla- or hazelnut-flavored coffee or a regular brew.)

1 cup strong mocha-flavored coffee (cold or hot)

1¼ cups fat-free milk

½ teaspoon orange extract

1 teaspoon sugar or honey (optional)

Unsweetened cocoa powder

In a pitcher, combine the coffee, milk, orange extract, and sugar or honey, if using. Stir. Serve hot or iced. Dust with cocoa powder before serving. Makes two 1½-cup servings.

FAQs for Phase 4

Q: *I love my energy bars, but they tend to contain a lot of added sugars. How can I make a smart choice?*

Now that you're free to enjoy 6 to 9 teaspoons (24 to 36 grams) of added sugars a day in any way your sugary little heart desires, you'll want to keep track of how many grams you're consuming.

Sometimes, "sugar math" is easy. Stir a teaspoon of the sweet stuff into your coffee or drizzle a teaspoon of honey on your morning oatmeal, and you've consumed 4 grams of sugar, or one-sixth of your daily allotment. But as I've mentioned before, determining the amount of added sugars in packaged or prepared foods can be tricky. Food manufacturers aren't required to separate naturally occurring and added sugars on their labels. What they list is the product's total sugars, which can come from the sugars naturally in the food, added sugars, or both.

Sneaky! But not sneaky enough. Here's a quick-and-dirty way to estimate any food's added sugars.

- On the product's Nutrition Facts label, look for Total Sugars.
- If the product contains 0 grams of sugar (or a minimal amount, say up to 3 grams), you're in the clear.
- If the product contains sugar, consider all of it to be added unless the food contains a significant

Sweet Freedom Strategy: Indulge in Some Fragrant "Tub Therapy"

Stressed and achy from a long day of desk-jockeying? Get in the tub and turn a ho-hum soak into a spa-like pleasure. But the water's got to be *hot*.

At first, hot baths raise your heart rate and temperature, says *Prevention* advisory board member Tieraona Low Dog, MD. To dispel that heat, you perspire, which allows your body to rid itself of toxins. Then your blood vessels dilate and increase circulation, removing lactic acid from muscles, lowering blood pressure, and easing pain.

amount of fruit, milk, or yogurt, or "sweeter" vegetables such as beets, carrots, corn, green peas, sweet potatoes, and winter squash.

- Look at the product's ingredients list. Do you spot any form of added sugar? No? Then the sugar is naturally present in the food. Two examples: plain yogurt and unsweetened applesauce.

- If you do spot sugar or its aliases, it's sugar math time. Don't get nervous. Once you're familiar with how much natural sugar unsweetened foods contain, it's a snap to guesstimate how much added sugar the sweetened versions are packing.

For example, ½ cup of frozen corn has 4 grams of sugar but just one ingredient: corn. The same amount of canned cream-style corn contains 7 grams of sugar. Check the ingredients list—sure enough, sugar is listed. So you can figure that the canned variety has about 3 grams of added sugar. Or take unsweetened versus sweetened applesauce—12 grams of sugar for the unsweetened versus 25 grams per ½ cup for the sweetened (thanks, high-fructose corn syrup!). Do you love cream-style corn enough to spend almost a whole teaspoon of sugar on it? Do you want applesauce to supply nearly half your daily allowance of added sugar? It's your choice. But thanks to sugar math, you have one.

Here's Dr. Low Dog's recipe for a detox bath. To a tub of hot water, add 2 tablespoons of sea salt and 10 drops of one of the essential oils below, which you can pick up at any natural foods store.

To tame tension, try clary sage. The wonderful floral aroma relaxes you and lifts your spirits.

When you feel frazzled, luxuriate in lavender. This lovely floral fragrance helps ground and center you. It's perfect for those days when you're feeling anxious.

Reconsidering Your Key Sugar Source

Reunited and it feels so good: In Phase 4, you can reintroduce the key sugar source you identified during Countdown, along with your other sugary favorites. How do you feel about this? Excited? A bit anxious about sliding back into old patterns?

It's time to find out. Based on the "eating with mindfulness" strategy from Chapter 7, the exercise below can help you assess the previous role your key sugar source and other favorite treats played in your life, and decide what part they will play in the future. You'll need a small portion of your key sugar source and 5 minutes in a quiet spot without distractions.

1. Put a small portion on a plate. If possible, sit at your kitchen table.

2. Consider your treat. Recall what you liked about it and the feelings it brought up, positive or negative, when you ate it. Compare those feelings to the way you've been feeling since it's been out of your diet. How do you think having the treat might change that? Are you looking forward to your first bite? What do you expect to feel after you eat it?

3. Take a bite, being mindful of its flavor and texture. Does it taste the way you remember? Are you getting a rush of pleasure?

4. Finish the treat, continuing to eat slowly and mindfully. Do you still love it? Did you miss it? Would you still consider it your key sugar source?

5. When you're done, ponder these questions: Did the treat live up to your expectations? Do you want more now, or are you satisfied with the small portion you had? Would you have been just as satisfied with another food?

6. Over the next hour, monitor your body and feelings carefully. Are you hungry sooner than you might have been otherwise? Do you feel cravings for more of your key sugar source, or another sugary food? Do you feel headachy or fatigued? Or do you feel good physically and pleased that you treated yourself to something you love?

To calm and clear your mind, soak in sandalwood. Its warm, woodsy scent has been used for centuries to prepare the mind for meditation. Check the

Before you started this plan, you may have turned to sugary foods out of habit or to soothe negative emotions. Or you may have been caught up in a cycle of sugar highs and lows that drove you to reach for more sugar. But now that you've broken the habit, found other ways to cope with stress, and stabilized your metabolism, where does your key sugar source fit in?

- **It still satisfies.** Then have it—but in a reasonable way. If you can limit yourself to a small portion with 100 to 150 calories, then you can have it every day in place of the dessert options in this phase. (If you want bigger serving sizes, wait until after Phase 4 and read the advice beginning on page 218.)

- **It's not as pleasurable, but I still want some sugary treats in my life.** Try some of the quick and healthy dessert options in this phase. They may be all you need now.

- **Overall, it's lost most of its allure.** Then why eat it? Many of our panelists found their perfect balance in either Phase 2 or 3. If that sounds like you, stick to that phase until you change your mind—if you ever do.

- **It still triggers cravings, hunger, or other symptoms.** Consider replacing your key sugar source with other sweets and carefully monitor your feelings and reactions. If any dessertlike food seems to have the same effect, stay on Phase 3 for another 2 weeks, then try again.

You might think about repeating this exercise with other favorite treats to gauge your reactions to them. There are no right or wrong answers; the purpose is to help raise your awareness of sugar's effects on you.

water temperature for comfort, then soak for 20 to 30 minutes. If you're pregnant or have heart problems, talk to your doctor before taking a detox bath.

LIVE THE SWEET LIFE FOR GOOD! SIX WAYS TO KEEP THE SUGAR FREEDOM FLOWING

As you prepare to strike out on your own, team the techniques you've used to manage stress and cravings throughout the plan with these big-picture strategies. Together, they'll help you stick to–and love–the sweet life.

1. Keep setting those daily intentions.

I hope that setting an intention has become a habit, one that's had a real impact on your life. Don't stop just because you've reached the end of the plan. Besides helping you to prioritize your health, intentions can steer you toward other goals and accomplishments.

My quiet time in the morning has helped me stay focused and even serene through some tough times, including moving three kids, two cats, two mice, three fish, and a frog to a new city and a new house while holding down a demanding job. Whether I use that time to meditate or merely to daydream, it's my oasis of calm where I turn down the volume on the competing demands on my energy and attention and focus on my personal priorities. When I set my daily intention, it's a pleasure to get out of bed to start the day. Hopefully, you've discovered that for yourself!

2. Always make time for your morning meal.

Metabolism revver. Brain booster. Cravings crusher. Breakfast is all of those things. So whether you've lost the weight you want or are still working on it, continue to eat breakfast each day, and make sure it contains 15 to 20 grams of lean protein. Feel free to enjoy your favorite breakfasts from any phase, and stock your refrigerator, freezer, and pantry with cravings-crushing breakfast ingredients like all-natural peanut butter, egg whites, low-fat ricotta cheese, and bags of frozen edamame.

3. Splurge once a week.

It's your birthday or someone else's, and there is cake. You're visiting the town with the best ice cream shop on the planet. You're at a restaurant where the desserts are to die for. Or you just want a nice glass of lemonade on a hot summer day. I don't want you to concern yourself with parceling out a portion of the sugary treat that has exactly 150 calories and 12 grams of added sugar. Just have it—as long as you splurge only one time a week and skip your daily 150-calorie indulgence that day. The first few times, carefully monitor how you feel physically and emotionally afterward. Sometimes, the day after I've had an anything-goes meal is when I experience intense sugar cravings. Plan ahead, indulge, enjoy—and then clear your system of that sugar load by following a Phase 1 or 2 diet that day and perhaps even the next.

4. Stay ahead of "sugar creep."

When people on diet plans relax their eating, the result is "sugar creep." A gummy worm here, a few chips there—eventually, their nibbles and sips snowball, and they find themselves in a carb coma, wondering what happened.

What happened was that they stopped eating with awareness. Little by little, the healthy habits they worked so hard to integrate into their lives slipped away, and old habits took over. It doesn't have to happen to you. Here are three simple ways to outsmart sugar creep. Stick to them and you'll continue to enjoy all of the pleasures of sugar, with none of the drawbacks.

Keep reading labels. That positive habit reinforces awareness, and it can help snap you back to reality when you're considering a treat that you may not really want and didn't plan to enjoy. Say, for example, your partner brings home a boxed raspberry cheese Danish. The label says that one serving packs 15 grams of sugar. That's just short of 4 teaspoons—most of your daily allotment if you're a woman! Do you really want that slice? Or would a few squares of dark chocolate or a slice of whole grain toast with 100% raspberry spread hit the spot just as well?

Plan your indulgences. For the most part, you should decide what you'll have as a treat on any particular day and stick to that. If you don't know what you'll be in the mood for, at least determine ahead of time when you'll have sugar. Are you going out to dinner and want dessert? Do you plan on working hard through the afternoon and think a 4:00 p.m. treat will be a nice break? The idea is to limit your spontaneous sugar indulgences as much as possible. Planning not only helps you manage your intake of sugar but increases your enjoyment of it when you do indulge.

Always mind your first bite. Any time you have a sugary treat, give your full attention to the first bite. Gaze at it lovingly. Give thanks for it. Appreciate its color, scent, temperature, and complexity of flavors. It's a way to pay respect to sugar and keep your awareness of its presence in your diet sharp.

5. Have a plan for backsliding.

What if, despite your best intentions, sugar does creep up on you? Simply go back to Phase 1 for a week or two to reset your sugar thermostat. You can then either progress through the plan in the same way you just did or come straight back to Phase 4.

6. Savor life as much as sugar.

Take a moment to think about your schedule. Does it include an activity that puts a curl in your toes? The more pleasure and joy and laughter you add to your life, the less you'll feel the need to derive pleasure from food.

Years ago, a boyfriend's mother told me her secret to a fulfilling life: She did something she really loved for 20 minutes every day. This "20-minute rule" clicked with me, and I immediately made a list of nonfood pleasures that I could choose from as a reward.

In other words, hang on to your Rewards Card. Treat yourself to one of its pleasures each day, and as you discover new ones, revise your card. And remember—the sweetness of life is in the moment, and pleasure-filled moments make a life.

But there's another, lesser-known dimension to pleasure: *savoring*. To savor something is to enjoy it thoroughly, wringing every drop of pleasure from it. And research suggests it's the key to true happiness.

In a study published in the *Journal of Positive Psychology*, researchers had 101 women and men keep diaries for 30 days. They recorded "pleasant events" and how much they savored or squelched them. Savorers got more pleasure by stopping to focus on a good thing, telling someone else about it, or even screaming in delight. Wet-blanket types killed the joy by carping that it could have been better, they didn't deserve it, or it was almost over. Ultimately, savorers got the biggest happiness boost from pleasurable moments.

To reap the benefits of this little-known component of pleasure, embark on what the study's lead researcher calls a savoring adventure. It could be a walk in the woods, a trip into a city, or cooking a meal you love. Then do three things.

- Before the experience, anticipate how wonderful it will be.
- During the experience, focus on the sensations and feelings you're having. Use all five senses. Be nonjudgmental. Express your emotions to whomever you're with or by writing them down later.
- Afterward, look back on the event. Share it with someone.

Whatever your savor-worthy activity, start planning it now. Sugar is one of life's pleasures, and there are plenty more to revel in!

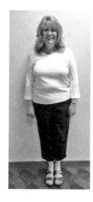

Debi Davies

For Debi, a Bible study fellowship teaching leader and education consultant, the Sugar Smart Plan was an educational opportunity for both her and her family. "I try to offer my teenage daughters healthy options," she says. "Now I recognize that what I was bringing into the house, packaged as healthy, such as granola bars and yogurt, wasn't so healthy."

As soon as Debi understood why certain changes were important, she was committed and didn't cheat. The first order of business was to clean out the snack drawer. While they didn't throw the food out, they put it in a bin and stored it out of the kitchen so Debi wasn't tempted and the girls and her husband ate less. Instead, they snack on the nuts and seeds that now fill the snack drawer.

"I tried to cut out artificial sweeteners when I heard that they can cause you to crave more sugar," says Debi, who replaced her diet soda with flavored seltzer. "I like carbonation, and it made me feel like I wasn't being 100 percent deprived."

When she learned that 4 grams of sugar equal a teaspoon, and that women shouldn't have more than 6 teaspoons of sugar a day, "that little bit of information really changed how I look at things," says Debi. She is reading labels and choosing foods with the lowest amounts of added sugar. "Do you know how hard it is to find a tomato sauce without added sugar? I went to five grocery stores to find one—and then I brought home several jars." They haven't given up their beloved ketchup, but they do use less of it and of salad dressings.

Debi's oldest daughter makes batches of the energy bars from the original Sugar Smart Diet. Another family treat has been creations from a Yonanas machine that makes yummy "ice cream" from frozen fruit. "We put more thought into what we're eating," she says, adding that her husband has lost weight, too. "This weekend, we were at two events where candy was everywhere in front of me. Afterward, my husband said, 'I can't believe you didn't have one piece of licorice.' It's about being more mindful about what I'm eating versus eating just because I can."

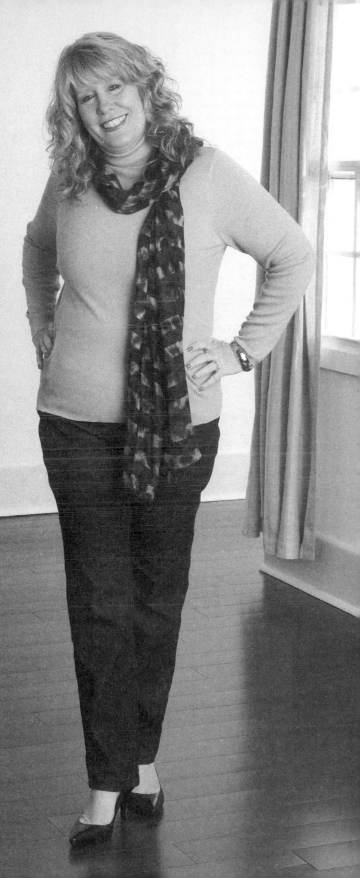

5.1
POUNDS LOST

AGE:
48

ALL-OVER INCHES LOST:
6.75

SUGAR SMART WISDOM:
"The longer you cook a sweet potato, the sweeter it gets. I now cook mine for about 2 hours and eat it plain because it's so sweet."

Dining Out and Special Occasions

Eat Sugar-Smart Anytime, Anywhere

My family and I eat most of our meals at home. Even so, there always seems to be an on-the-go meal, a planned dinner at our favorite restaurant, or a special occasion. You too? No surprise there–the average American dines out four to five times a week, according to the National Restaurant Association.

But *any* time you nosh away from home–burger joint, Chinese place, party, wedding–your sugary spidey sense should tingle. *Especially* if you're dining at a chain restaurant. Between the huge portions and the carefully cultivated "live a little, eat a lot!" vibe, chains can be sugar-bomb minefields.

Recently, the Center for Science in the Public Interest (CSPI) handed out its annual awards for the unhealthiest meals at fast-food and chain restaurants. In horror, I read that the single unhealthiest meal the CSPI tested–Red Robin's Gourmet "Monster"-Sized A.1. Peppercorn Burger, Bottomless Steak Fries, and Monster Salted Caramel Milkshake–packed an estimated $3/_4$ cup of added sugar. That's nearly 36 teaspoons. In one meal. (The calorie, fat, and sodium numbers were just as terrifying. Whoever came up with this food-mare is the Stephen King of chain-restaurant menus.)

I don't have jeans big enough for that kind of sugar-soaked fare. So when I eat away, I ask myself a simple question that helps me decide when to indulge in sugar and carbs, and when to pass them up.

Is this food really, truly, mind-blowingly special?

Special, as in: *It's my favorite. I can only have it at this place, and I'm here twice a year, tops. Only Mom makes it this good. This is a bona fide occasion, and this food or drink will add to my pleasure.*

If it's truly amazingly special, I indulge–a little. A bite or two of the to-die-for *gâteau* at my favorite restaurant. Brunch with friends, where one orange mimosa sweetens the jazz. My aunt's secret-recipe potato salad. Just like identifying your personal where, when, and why (Chapter 6), asking this question ensures that you *enjoy* sugar, not just consume it.

For such special meals, I also have a plan. More than likely, I know what I'll have before I even get there. On special occasions, when food and company are equally pleasurable, that plan helps me focus on the celebrating or socializing rather than the dessert table.

Went to Outback this weekend and had a grilled sirloin, a sweet potato (no brown sugar!), and grilled asparagus. My meal was good and I felt like there were enough options to choose from. My husband ordered the brownie sundae. I was a little jealous but felt satisfied in terms of fullness. —Joelle

Because of our crazy-busy lives, eating away often is about convenience (or exhaustion). But sometimes it's truly special. When you're sugar smart, you're aware of the difference and free to make choices that protect your health, shrink your sugar belly–and taste divine. This chapter reveals the best low-sugar menu options at 10 top restaurant and pizza chains and shows you how to choose flavor over sugar when you head out for ethnic cuisine. But first, some dining-out ground rules. Stick to them, and you're ahead of the sugar game before you even put your napkin on your lap.

NO-BRAINER SUGAR SLASHERS

You already know the low-fat drill. Select grilled, roasted, or broiled fare over fried. Skip the sauces and gravies. Say, "Hold the butter and oil, please." Those old-timey tips will always be in vogue–they can help cut sugar as well as fat. But you have even more sugar-slashing tools to use when you dine out. In some cases, you can limit your sugar consumption before you even pick up the menu.

Plan for splurges. Remember I said I had a plan? This is part of what I meant, a basic technique for when you know what's on the menu or at the event. If you're dying for the cheesecake at your favorite restaurant, follow Phase 1 the day before your meal and bank your sugar allotment. The same recommendation applies when you know you'll want a slice of cake at a wedding, or Aunt Emily's signature holiday dish.

"Order" online before you go. Not familiar with the restaurant? Get thee to Google–most restaurants post their menus online. Review the menu online the day before, make your low-sugar selections, and decide what you'll order. Once seated, don't even open the menu–just rattle off your order. If you can ask for a party or holiday menu in advance, adopt a similar strategy. That way, you're not overwhelmed by the choices on the table or at the buffet.

BYOD. Remember, low-calorie or low-fat salad dressings are typically loaded with sugar! Those offered at most restaurants can turn even a

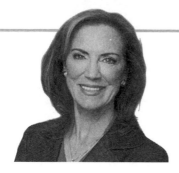

Sweet Inspiration

Pam Peeke, MD, MPH, FACP

Know your "sugar saturation point." Refined or processed sugar is ubiquitous in our food. As a result, the brain's reward center is constantly being ignited, stirring up an endless appetite for these empty calories. In vulnerable individuals, consuming refined and processed sugar to excess results in an addictive process. If someone has a high level of sugar addiction, the intake should be very minimal. The key is to know how much of which food will trigger a feeling of loss of control and overeating or a binge. For instance, a regular chocolate bar with a high level of refined sugar is too much for most people and may result in overeating. However, an organic bar with at least 70 percent cacao may not, as it has so much less sugar. The source of sugar is important.

Customize your cut-sugar strategy. There are a number of ways to cut back on sugar. You can wean yourself—for example, from six sugar sodas down, then on to diet sodas, then to seltzer water, and finally to plain water perhaps flavored with lemon or orange slices. But if you are addicted to the stuff, an immediate detox may be necessary for you to break free and stop caving to the craving. Increasing physical activity is wonderful to help regulate appetite and hunger. So is getting 7 to 8 hours of high-quality sleep.

Try a protein-fiber craving killer. The only time I crave refined sugar is when I'm stressed out. When that toxic stress hits, there's an instant urge to grab something sweet. It's like a knee-jerk reaction. At that very moment, I'll grab something with protein and fiber that will kill the craving. Peanut or almond butter on a piece of fruit like apple slices or a banana works well, as does yogurt with walnuts and berries.

Take out "sugar insurance" against cravings. As a preemptive strike against sugar cravings, I meditate twice a day for 20 minutes each time. Meditation increases your ability to draw upon your prefrontal cortex (the CEO of the brain) to stay vigilant and make the right decisions.

PAM PEEKE, MD, MPH, FACP, is assistant clinical professor of medicine at the University of Maryland. An internationally renowned expert on nutrition, metabolism, stress, and fitness, she is the author of *Body for Life for Women, Fight Fat after Forty,* and *Fit to Live.* Her most recent book is *The Hunger Fix: The Three-Stage Detox and Recovery Plan for Overeating and Food Addiction.*

grilled-chicken salad into a sugar bomb. Don't let dressings do you in. If you opt for a dinner-size salad, either stick to a basic oil and vinegar dressing or–if you're brave–bring along your favorite low-sugar bottled dressing. Chances are, neither your waiter nor the other patrons will bat an eye.

Practice proactive portion control. I don't need to tell you that restaurant portions are notoriously huge. But this tip can save you: Ask your server to serve just half of your meal and box up the other half to take home.

Keep your mind on your meal. Who says you can't savor a tasty restaurant meal *and* practice the principles of mindful eating? In a small study published in the *Journal of Nutrition Education and Behavior,* older women who ate away from home at least three times a week, but who practiced mindful eating while dining out, lost almost 4 pounds in 6 weeks, even though they were only trying to maintain their weight. They also ate fewer calories and grams of fat per day, and they found it easier to manage their weight. If you're too bashful to use the tip above, mindful eating will help you stop when you're full, not when your plate is clean.

THE SUGAR SMART EXPRESS DINING-OUT MENU: SIMPLE, SCRUMPTIOUS, LOW-SUGAR FARE

Maybe you think sit-down restaurants are healthier than fast-food places. Not necessarily, according to a 2014 study of more than 12,000 adults, published in the journal *Public Health Nutrition.* On days these folks ate out, the study found, they consumed roughly 200 extra calories, whether they ate at fast-food joints or full-service restaurants. Worse, the typical American consumes an extra 24,000 calories a year by eating out, the study estimated–the equivalent of 6 to 7 pounds a year.

Ouch. But now that you've acquired sugar smarts, you're free to order a meal that's low in added sugars anywhere. Simply follow the template on page 230, and your healthy meal will build itself. (Of course, you don't have to order everything on the "menu.")

The Express Menu

BROTH-BASED SOUP OR STEAMED SEAFOOD

Steamed clams or shrimp cocktail, minus the sugary cocktail sauce

SALAD DRESSED WITH BALSAMIC VINEGAR AND OLIVE OIL

For a touch of sweet or crunch, you may add

1 tablespoon dried fruit or 1 tablespoon of nuts or seeds if desired.

LEAN PROTEIN–BEEF, FISH, POULTRY, OR PORK

Choose lean cuts, prepared without butter or fatty sauces.

Poaching in wine adds flavor, but the sugar is burned off during cooking.

GRILLED, ROASTED, OR STEAMED VEGETABLES

1 to 2 cups, prepared without fatty sauces
(1 teaspoon butter optional on steamed veggies only)

WHOLE GRAIN OR POTATO*

1 cup cooked brown rice or other grain, plain or with 1 pat butter, if desired
or 1 small or ½ large baked potato, plain or with 1 pat butter, lemon, and
pepper if desired

No whole grain/starchy vegetable options? Increase protein to 8 ounces.

FRUIT FOR DESSERT

For example, a poached pear, a bowl of fresh berries,
a half-cup of fruit salad

Optional: One 5-ounce glass of wine or one 12-ounce glass of beer or
one shot of spirits in a sugar-free mixer, enjoyed with dinner,
rather than before dinner

10 TOP EATERIES, 50 SUGAR SMART OPTIONS

Hungry? Get ready to enjoy a healthy, low-sugar meal at one of your favorite fast-food or chain restaurants—without feeling hungry or deprived. To maximize deliciousness and minimize sugar, keep a few things in mind.

1. The items listed represent the best that each restaurant has to offer. Pass up known sugar bombs—desserts, sodas, shakes, smoothies.
2. All items listed are the smallest sizes available.
3. At big chain restaurants, appetizers are guilty until proven innocent.

Arby's

Jr. Roast Beef
Calories 210
Fiber 1 g
Sugars 4 g

Prime-Cut Chicken Tenders (3 Pieces)
Calories 350
Fiber 2 g
Sugars 0 g

Ham, Egg, and Cheese Wrap
Calories 420
Fiber 2 g
Sugars 1 g

Chopped Farmhouse Salad— Roast Turkey
Calories 230
Fiber 3 g
Sugars 4 g

Roast Beef Classic
Calories 360
Fiber 1 g
Sugars 6 g

Special Occasions: Think SLIM

Does any social event or celebration—from a simple dinner for two to a cocktail party or company picnic—ratchet up your appetite or turbocharge your sweet tooth? If so, I can relate. Parties used to present dual temptations: all-you-can-eat foods from the sugar-heaven list and opportunities for anonymous eating. (Who's going to notice if you scarf handfuls of cookies?)

But if you make a plan, social eating doesn't have to derail your progress. The low-sugar guidelines and emotional coping strategies below are easy to remember because they spell out the word SLIM. Review them before your next social event and remember them while you're there. More than likely, they'll help you stifle the impulse to wade into the chocolate fountain.

S: Stick to flavor, not sugar. If you're dining out, follow the advice in Chapter 11. At other events, stick to whole foods as much as possible, skipping sweetened beverages, slow-cooker fare, and store-bought pasta salad and macaroni salad. If you know the menu will offer mostly unhealthy options, eat one of your favorite meals from any of the phases before you go and then skip to the next letter on this list.

L: Love the ones you're with. The key to making it through a special occasion is to keep your focus on the celebration, rather than the food. When you attend an event where food will be served, make it a point to talk to at least one person—your favorite aunt at a family reunion, the coworker who shares your interest in hiking or gardening. The more attention you give to others, the less you'll give to the food.

Boston Market

Rotisserie Chicken (Quarter White, Skinless)

Calories 220

Fiber 0 g

Sugars 0 g

Rotisserie Chicken (Quarter White, with Skin)

Calories 320

Fiber 0 g

Sugars 1 g

I: Imbibe sensibly—sip one drink, max. The stress of a social event, or the flaring of family tensions during the holidays, may tempt you to drink one more glass of wine than is wise. Keep your head. Overdoing it on alcohol can lower your inhibitions. That leaves you vulnerable to scarfing sugary treats at a party or ordering dessert when you hadn't planned to.

M: Monitor what you're thinking and feeling. During the event, notice any thoughts and feelings that being there brings up. Do you feel overwhelmed or shy? Overjoyed and ready to party? Intense emotion, negative or positive, can lead to overeating. To help keep you centered, practice one of the emotional coping strategies you've learned, both before and during the event.

Work the Room, Not the Food

In the publishing business, I attend a fair amount of events—book launches, media lunches, and the like. The one thing I can always count on: There will be food, and it will be (mostly) amazing.

Now that I'm sugar smart, however, I know how to handle these food-centric occasions. Gone are the days when I'd scarf finger foods or bonbons hand over fist. Today, I take my time perusing the hors d'oeuvres table or dessert tray, choosing the *one* item that blows my hair back, flavor-wise, and splurging on one serving. (I'm this choosy at weddings and non-work-related events, too.)

I also put my focus on catching up with old friends and meeting new ones. I've noticed that when I put people first—whether I'm working the room or having a heart-to-heart—it's easier to ignore the siren call of sugar.

Turkey Breast (Regular)

Calories 200

Fiber 0 g

Sugars 0 g

Garlic Dill New Potatoes

Calories 100

Fiber 2 g

Sugars 1 g

Fresh Steamed Vegetables

Calories 70

Fiber 3 g

Sugars 2 g

Carrabba's

Wood-Grilled Salmon (6 Ounces)

Calories 478

Fiber 0 g

Sugars 1 g

Wood-Grilled Chicken (Small)

Calories 179

Fiber 0 g

Sugars 0 g

Chicken Bryan (Small)

Calories 421

Fiber 0 g

Sugars 1 g

Minestrone Soup (Cup)

Calories 118

Fiber 5 g

Sugars 0 g

Caesar Salad (Side)

Calories 307

Fiber 3 g

Sugars 2 g

Chili's

6-Ounce Classic Sirloin

Calories 300

Fiber 0 g

Sugars 0 g

Grilled Chicken Salad

Calories 430

Fiber 5 g

Sugars 11 g

Rice and Black Beans

Calories 270

Fiber 7 g

Sugars 2 g

Chipotle Black Bean Burger Only

Calories 190

Fiber 8 g

Sugars 2 g

Parmesan-Crusted Tilapia

Calories 600

Fiber 8 g

Sugars 2 g

Papa John's

Papa's Chkn Poppers (5 Poppers)

Calories 180

Fiber 1 g

Sugars 0 g

Spicy Buffalo Wings (2 Pieces)

Calories 170

Fiber 0 g

Sugars 1 g

BBQ Wings (2 Pieces)

Calories 190

Fiber 0 g

Sugars 2 g

Cheese Pizza, Pizza for One (1 Slice)

Calories 180

Fiber 1 g

Sugars 3 g

Pepperoni Pizza, Pizza for One (1 Slice)

Calories 210

Fiber 1 g

Sugars 3 g

On my birthday, instead of a cake, my kind coworkers brought fresh fruit! I spent my birthday weekend in New York City. I had a grilled-chicken salad for lunch and fish, steamed veggies, and half a baked potato for dinner. Between meals, I had my snacks—yes, I took them with me. I found it easier to make good choices because I knew I was accountable for them. —Robin

Pizza Hut

Baked Wings, Naked (2 Pieces)

Calories 100

Fiber 0 g

Sugars 0 g

12-Inch Medium Pan Pizza, Cheese (1 Slice)

Calories 240

Fiber 1 g

Sugars 1 g

12-Inch Medium Pan Pizza, Pepperoni (1 Slice)

Calories 260

Fiber 1 g

Sugars 1 g

12-Inch Medium Hand-Tossed Pizza, Cheese (1 Slice)

Calories 210

Fiber 1 g

Sugars 1 g

12-Inch Medium Hand-Tossed Pizza, Pepperoni (1 Slice)

Calories 220

Fiber 1 g

Sugars 1 g

Quiznos

Basil Pesto Chicken Flatbread

Calories 360

Fiber 4 g

Sugars 5 g

Turkey, Ranch, and Swiss Sub

Calories 470

Fiber 3 g

Sugars 6 g

Ham and Egg Grilled Flatbread (Small)

Calories 300

Fiber 1 g

Sugars 5 g

Veggie Guacamole Sub

Calories 450

Fiber 3 g

Sugars 5 g

Chili (with 2 Crackers)

Calories 180

Fiber 3 g

Sugars 4 g

Smokey Bones Bar & Fire Grill

Fresh Steamed Broccoli

Calories 70

Fiber 3 g

Sugars 0 g

Caesar Side Salad

Calories 370

Fiber 2 g

Sugars 1 g

Chicken Fingers Appetizer

Calories 420

Fiber 2 g

Sugars 2 g

7-Ounce Top Sirloin (Mushroom Sauce)

Calories 420

Fiber 1 g

Sugars 2 g

Vegetable Burger

Calories 380

Fiber 8 g

Sugars 6 g

Sonic

Jr. Burger

Calories 330

Fiber 1 g

Sugars 3 g

Jr. Deluxe Burger

Calories 360

Fiber 1 g

Sugars 4 g

Jr. Breakfast Burrito

Calories 280

Fiber 0 g

Sugars 0 g

Super Crunch Chicken Strips (3 Pieces)

Calories 330

Fiber 2 g

Sugars 0 g

Tots (Small)

Calories 220

Fiber 2 g

Sugars 0 g

Tony Roma's

Norwegian Salmon— Blackened or Grilled

Calories 536

Fiber 2 g

Sugars 0 g

Filet Medallions—Asiago Crust

Calories 348

Fiber 0 g

Sugars 0 g

Dinner Caesar Side Salad

Calories 215

Fiber 2 g

Sugars 3 g

Chicken Spinach Stack (Includes Wild Rice Blend)

Calories 594

Fiber 2 g

Sugars 3 g

Chipotle Sausage and Roasted Vegetable Soup (Cup)

Calories 150

Fiber 1 g

Sugars 4 g

"Where's My Favorite Restaurant?"

You may be wondering why this chapter doesn't list some of your favorite restaurant chains. It's because a fair number of national chains don't list sugar values in their nutritional information.

These restaurants include:

Applebee's
Baja Fresh
The Cheesecake Factory
Olive Garden
Panera Bread
Red Lobster
Ruby Tuesday
TGI Friday's

Two national chains didn't offer nutritional information at all: Cracker Barrel and Texas Roadhouse.

Take heart—you don't have to avoid these restaurants. Simply follow the "menu" on page 230 to order a meal that fits the Express guidelines. Or use the interactive nutrition calculators offered by some restaurant chains like Chipotle Mexican Grill and Red Robin. They're fun to use, and more important, they teach you how to make sugar smart choices.

For example, Red Robin's online "Customizer" allows you to plug in the item on the menu you'd like to eat; then, the application calculates its nutrition values and allows you to add or omit ingredients. For example, a Simply Grilled Chicken Salad contains 539 calories, 8 grams of sugar, 6 grams of fiber, and 46 grams of protein. Omit the cheese, and your meal lightens up to 428 calories, with no changes to sugar and fiber.

Using Chipotle's calculator, you can build your own taco, burrito, burrito bowl, or salad, and it's entirely possible to build a healthy meal. For example, a taco on a soft corn tortilla with chicken, fajita veggies, and salsa contains 440 calories, 6 grams of sugar, and 5 grams of fiber. *Muy delicioso!*

Colleen DiRosa

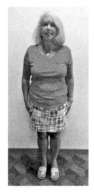

The Sugar Smart Express Plan helped Colleen get back on a healthy track—and just in the nick of time.

Colleen had always been active, playing tennis and working out at the gym regularly. She was an avid skier, and her family took frequent active vacations centered around hiking or biking. But in the past 2 years, despite all of her activity, she started to gain weight. As a result, "my joints, especially my knees, started hurting, and I felt sluggish," Colleen says. "I remember thinking that I shouldn't be huffing and puffing so much on a hilly bike ride."

Last winter, this lifelong skier, who had raced in college, had to cut back on her skiing. "I couldn't do moguls because it hurt too much. I had turned into this old lady," she says.

Things got worse last April when one of Colleen's best friends passed away. "My whole life fell apart," she says. "I stopped exercising, ate more junk, and gained more weight."

As her grieving subsided, Colleen was ready to take back control of her life. Little did she know how valuable the Sugar Smart Plan was going to be when she signed up. Shortly after Colleen completed the 3-week plan, her 16-year-old daughter was diagnosed with diabetes. "When it happened, I was like, 'I can handle this,' instead of falling apart," she says, attributing her confidence to the knowledge she had gained from her experience. "I was able to teach her a whole new way of eating like I had just learned."

In addition to finding out how to get sugar—especially Sugar Mimics like pretzels and bread that Colleen craved—out of her diet, Colleen also finally canceled her membership in the clean plate club. "I grew up with the philosophy that you had to finish what's on your plate all the time," she says. But at her 25th wedding anniversary party, she had just a few bites of the delicious peanut butter raspberry cake. "I was satisfied. I realized that I don't have to eat the whole thing."

Colleen's success on the program also inspired her to hire a personal trainer. With a stepped-up exercise program and slimmer figure, Colleen has found that her knees are no longer achy—and she's looking forward to hitting the slopes this winter. "Last year, my kids were calling me 'old.' I'm going to show them. I'm not going to be such a wuss!"

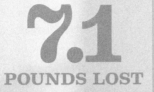

7.1
POUNDS LOST

AGE:
47

**ALL-OVER
INCHES LOST:**
6.75

**SUGAR SMART
WISDOM:**
*"Sprinkle a peach or
pear with cinnamon
and bake it in the
toaster oven for a
sweet treat reminis-
cent of yummy cobbler
or pie."*

LOW-SUGAR ETHNIC CHOICES

I adore ethnic food. Italian, French, Asian, Middle Eastern, Mexican–you name it, I eat it. But my all-time favorite is Indian cuisine. Something about those warming spices, from freshly grated ginger and turmeric to curry and cumin, just sucks me in. When I get on a curry jag, as I do now and again, I'll whip up curried pumpkin soup one night, curried chickpeas and brown rice the next, curried vegetable and lamb stew to savor on the weekend.

Most ethnic cuisine is healthy, I'm happy to report. Unfortunately, the way it's prepared in American restaurants may not be. To limit your sugar intake when you eat ethnic food, use the cheat sheet below. It offers a sampling of healthy options and terms to look for when making your selections, as well as sugar bombs to sidestep.

Chinese

- *Zheng* (steamed)
- *Jum* (poached)
- *Kao* (roasted)
- "Stock velveted" (cooked in seasoned water rather than oil)
- Brown rice, not white (or skip the rice entirely)
- Sugar bombs: General Tso's chicken; sweet-and-sour dishes; high-sugar duck, plum, and hoisin sauces

Greek/Middle Eastern

- Greek salad with lemon and oil dressing (request feta cheese and dressing on the side)
- *Plaki* (fish cooked in tomatoes and onions)
- Souvlaki or kebabs (marinated and broiled or grilled meat on a skewer with vegetables). Hold the rice.

- *Tabbouleh* (bulgur wheat salad with lemon and mint)
- Sugar bombs: baklava; moussaka (rich, creamy topping over ground meat and oily eggplant)

Indian

- Tandoor (chicken, meat, or fish cooked in a clay oven with spices)
- *Raita* (flavorful yogurt sauce)
- Vegetable curries prepared without *ghee* (clarified butter)
- Sugar bombs: chutney; fried breads such as *poori;* dishes made with coconut milk

Italian

- Red sauces
- Piccata (lemon)
- Mussels *fra diavolo* (tomato-based sauce spiced with chile peppers)
- Lightly sautéed
- Grilled
- Sugar bombs: pasta (the ultimate Sugar Mimic). Try a red sauce over steamed spinach or grilled veggies instead.

Japanese

- Broiled or grilled fish
- *Oshitoshi* (steamed spinach)
- Yakitori (grilled chicken)
- Sashimi
- Sugar bombs: rice (a Sugar Mimic); teriyaki sauce; soy sauce; yakitori sauce

Mexican

- *Ceviche* (fresh fish or shrimp marinated with lime juice)
- Rice and black beans
- Salsa or picante
- Soft corn tortillas
- Sugar bombs: chimichangas; flan

Thai

- Papaya salad
- Satay (skewer of grilled meat or poultry)
- Water-based curries (*gaeng pah*), which are prepared with water rather than coconut milk
- Sugar bombs: sweet coconut rice; dishes prepared with coconut milk or peanut sauces

The Express Workout: Mini but Mighty

Exercise is optional on the Sugar Smart Express Plan. That's right. You don't want to do it? You don't have to.

That said, you should totally do it. Just a little. And a little is all you need to help control your sugar cravings, manage your blood sugar levels, maintain the calorie-burning muscle you have, and maybe even help speed up your weight loss.

If you already have a workout routine you enjoy, stick with it! If not, here's the plan.

Most days of the week: Walk briskly for 30 minutes. Break up your walk into 10- or 15-minute segments, or not–it's up to you.

Two or 3 days a week: Zip through the Express Workout, developed by Michele Stanten, *Prevention*'s former fitness director, walking coach, and certified fitness instructor. You'll find the moves on page 252. And I do mean zip. We're talking three moves, at home, that should take you 15 minutes, max. All you need is a pair of dumbbells.

Maybe you're wondering, "Why on earth would I exercise if I don't have to? More drudgery in my life I don't need."

To which I reply: You're living the sweet life now. That means you're invited to change your perception of drudgery—and of rewards. You have nothing to lose but your sugar belly!

THE CASE FOR MOVING IT

Essayist and literary critic C. S. Lewis observed, "We are not bodies with souls, but rather souls with bodies." Exercise is a way to bring them together. In a very real sense, people who exercise regularly are tending their lives along with their bodies. We all know someone who raves about how her daily walk or run or gym time has changed her life. If you open your mind to the rewards of exercise that don't involve the scale, and seek pleasure in moving your body, that someone can be you.

I know this because this "rebranding" of exercise happened to me. Twenty years ago, punishment. Today, pleasure. What changed? My perspective! Today, exercise isn't about "fixing" jiggly bits; it's about spending quality time with me. I've also identified the exercises that feel good to me—yoga and fast walking outdoors—and do those, rather than force myself to do what doesn't feel good (running, trudging on the treadmill).

Still not convinced? What if I told you that the way you perceive exercise could make a difference in your desire for sugary, fatty treats? Well, it can, according to a series of studies conducted by the Food and Brand Lab at Cornell University in Ithaca, New York. (One of the researchers: Brian Wansink, PhD, who's spent most of his career studying the psychology behind what we eat—especially packaged food—and what makes us eat it.)

In one of the studies, researchers broke 56 women into two groups. Both groups went on a mile-long walk around a lake. But one group was told that they were engaged in an "exercise walk." The other group was told that the purpose of the walk was to do something fun. Plus, this group got to listen to music. (The exercise group got no tunes—only a map.)

After the groups finished walking, both received lunch. Those who'd gone on the "exercise walk" ate 35 percent more chocolate pudding for dessert than those who'd taken the "scenic walk." A second study of 46 women found that, compared to a "scenic walk" group, those who took the "exercise walk" ate 206 more calories of M&Ms—124 percent more!

In other words, view the *walk itself* as a reward. When you think, "What a gorgeous day!" rather than, "Almost done," you're less likely to "reward" yourself for hitting the walking path.

The bottom line? Commit to building fun and rewards into your workout. Listen to music. Select a scenic spot. Treat yourself to a sleek new pair of walking shoes or some pretty walking togs. Be grateful that you're in motion, instead of at the office. Before long you'll savor your workout, just as you've learned to savor your daily sugary treat. But you don't have to take my word for it. There's evidence that this is so.

Once you're in the right frame of mind—that "sweet spot," if you will—you're ready to move.

WALK THIS WAY

Brisk walking—and any activity that raises your heart rate, from cycling to Zumba class—helps melt the just-under-the-skin fluff that pads your hips, thighs, butt, chest, arms, and back. It keeps a sugar belly gone, too: Just 80 minutes a week slowed weight gain in 97 overweight women and stopped them from regaining visceral fat a year after weight loss, according to a study in the journal *Obesity*.

You can walk outside or use the stationary bike, treadmill, or elliptical trainer you have at home or at your gym. However, although walking is one of the simplest and most effective forms of fitness there is, it pays to do it right. Proper form can increase your speed, which will maximize your calorie burn. Each time you step outside, practice this checklist of proper techniques. If you're walking on a treadmill, the same techniques apply.

LOWER BODY

- Many people trying to walk briskly take overly long strides, which can actually slow you down. Instead, take shorter, quicker steps, rolling from heel to toes and pushing off with your toes.
- Keep your torso upright. Leaning too far forward or back will slow you down.
- It's okay for your waist to twist as you walk. Trying to reduce the movement of your hips will slow you down.

UPPER BODY

- Keep your head upright, your eyes straight ahead, and your shoulders and neck relaxed.
- Keep your elbows at 90 degrees and your hands relaxed.
- Swing your arms forward and back, and keep them close to your body.
- To increase your pace, speed up your arm swing. Your legs will follow!

STRENGTH-TRAINING BASICS

Three moves, 2 or 3 days a week. It doesn't get easier than this—and the benefits for such a brief workout couldn't be higher. When you lose weight, that loss is a combination of fat and calorie-burning muscle. But you don't want to lose muscle—that's what fuels your metabolism! Further, the stronger you are, the easier it is to move around and *keep* moving. This teensy routine can help minimize your muscle loss, so it'll be easier for you to lose additional weight and keep lost pounds lost.

If you're new to strength training, the Express Workout is a breeze.

Eat Dinner, Walk Off Diabetes Risk—In Just 15 Minutes

What's your typical after-dinner routine? If it involves your tablet or laptop, log off and lace up your sneakers instead. A 15-minute walk after the evening meal can help regulate blood sugar and reduce risk of type 2 diabetes, according to a study published in the journal *Diabetes Care*.

In this study, 10 healthy seniors spent three 48-hour spans in a lab. During each session, participants ate the same foods and followed one of three exercise routines: They either walked at an easy-to-moderate pace on a treadmill for 15 minutes after each meal, walked 45 minutes in the morning, or walked 45 minutes in the afternoon. In each of the three scenarios, the participants' blood sugar levels were tracked 24/7 with "continuous glucose monitoring," in which a tiny sensor inserted under the skin kept track of glucose levels.

The short postmeal walks were more effective at regulating blood sugar levels for up to 24 hours, the study found. This is key, because typically, your body can handle the normal blood sugar fluctuations that occur about 30 minutes after you eat. But as you get older (or if you're inactive throughout the day), your body doesn't react as efficiently, which leads to prolonged high blood sugar levels. The same thing happens if you are insulin sensitive or if you have diabetes. Over time, as you've learned, chronically high blood sugar can heighten your risk of getting type 2 diabetes and heart disease.

The exaggerated rise in blood sugar after the evening meal—often the largest of the day—can last well into the night and early morning. This was curbed significantly as soon as the volunteers hit the treadmill. In other words, if you're breaking your 30-minute walk into two segments, definitely get one in after dinner!

But just as with walking, proper form is crucial—you'll reap more benefits and avoid injury. The guidelines below cover proper form and breathing techniques. Keep in mind that it's normal to experience slight muscle soreness or fatigue. It should fade after a week or two.

- You'll need one set of dumbbells. If you're a beginner, we recommend starting with 3- and 5-pounders. If you're already lifting weights, try 5- and 8-pounders. However, keep in mind that the right weight for you may be heavier or lighter.

- The word *rep* is short for repetition. Each time you lift and lower a dumbbell, or roll your upper body up off the floor and then lower it back down, you've completed 1 repetition. A specific number of repetitions is called a set.

- The amount of weight you start with depends on how fit you are. But most people underestimate their strength and fitness level. If you can breeze through a set without fatigue, your weights are too light. The last rep should feel hard. If you can barely get through the last few reps of an exercise, though, you need a lighter weight. You may need different weight amounts for different exercises.

- Perform the moves slowly and with focus. Take 3 seconds to lift or push a weight into place, hold the position for 1 second, and take another 3 seconds to return to your starting position.

- Don't hold your breath. This can cause changes in blood pressure, especially for people with heart disease. Rather, inhale slowly through your nose and exhale slowly through your mouth.

- Exhale as you lift or push, and inhale as you relax.

- Use smooth, steady movements. To prevent injury, don't jerk or thrust weights into position, and avoid "locking" your knees and elbows.

- Don't perform the routine 2 days in a row. A day in between gives your muscles time to repair themselves—a necessary step for building strength.

Another Role for Exercise: Brain Fertilizer

Need another reason to hit the walking path more often? Exercise releases a "master molecule" in the brain that sharpens thinking, reduces stress, and improves mood, research has found.

A protein called BDNF—short for brain-derived neurotrophic factor—is known to promote the health of the 100 billion nerve cells (or neurons) in your brain, encouraging their growth and protecting them from stress. BDNF is "a crucial biological link between thought, emotions, and movement," says John J. Ratey, MD, associate clinical professor of psychiatry at Harvard Medical School.

Located in the hippocampus, the part of the brain associated with memory and learning, BDNF helps build and maintain the cellular circuitry in the brain and nourishes neurons as fertilizer feeds a growing plant. Sprinkled on neurons in a petri dish, BDNF causes them to sprout new branches, called dendrites.

Physical activity is the one clearly established way to raise levels of BDNF in the brain. Within minutes of your body getting moving, your brain perks up. Remember those studies about dopamine and pictures of milkshakes? Exercise sets off the brain's reward circuitry, which is why you see runners running in the pouring rain or 3 feet of snow.

Because BDNF is most active in the areas of the brain vital to learning, memory, and higher thinking, surges of the protein may contribute to why exercisers display sharper memory, higher concentration levels, and greater problem-solving skills than sedentary people. In a German study, volunteers who did two 3-minute sprints (separated by 2 minutes of lower intensity) during the course of a 40-minute treadmill session demonstrated higher increases in BDNF than non-sprinters. Plus, they learned vocabulary words 20 percent faster than non-sprinting men. Another study, on schoolchildren, found that 30 minutes on a treadmill improved performance on problem-solving exercises by 10 percent.

The Express Workout Moves

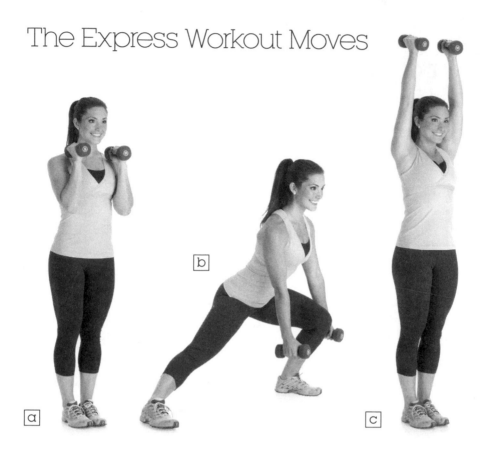

[a] [b] [c]

● Side Lunge with a Curl and Press

Stand with your feet together and hold the dumb-bells by your shoulders, arms bent and elbows pointing down **[a]**. Step your left foot out to the side and bend your left leg to sit back while keeping the right leg straight. As you lunge, extend your arms and lower the dumbbells **[b]**. Press into your left foot and straighten your leg to stand up. As you do that, bend your elbows and curl the dumb-bells toward your shoulders, then press them over-head as you bring your feet back together **[c]**. Do 10 times, then repeat the lunge on the opposite side.

Make it easier: Break up the exercise into two sepa-rate moves: Do the side lunges, only going as low as is comfortable for your knees. Then stand with your feet about hip-width apart and perform a biceps curl followed by an overhead press.

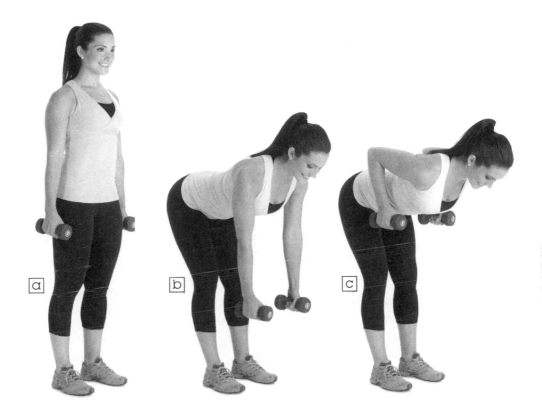

● Hinge and Row

Stand with your feet about hip-width apart, holding the dumbbells with your arms at your sides **[a]**. Keeping your abs tight and your chest lifted, bend at the hips and slowly lower until your torso is about parallel to the floor and the dumbbells hang beneath your shoulders **[b]**. Don't round your back. Bend your elbows and pull the dumbbells up toward your rib cage **[c]**. Lower the dumbbells and then stand back up. Do 10 times.

Make it easier: Do single-arm rows with a chair. Holding one dumbbell, bend forward and place your free hand on the seat of a chair, then perform rows with the opposite arm.

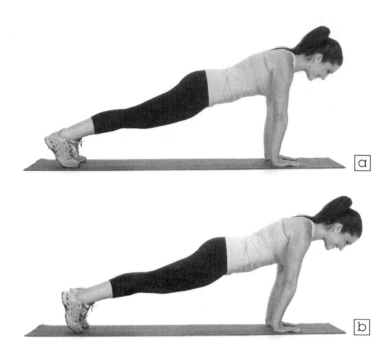

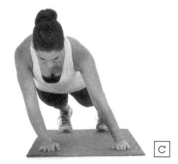

● Shifting Plank

Hold a pushup position, balancing on the balls of your feet and toes and your palms, hands directly beneath your shoulders **[a]**. Shift your weight forward **[b]**, to the left, and to the right **[c]**, without moving your hands. Hold each position for up to a count of 5 and return to center in between each shift. Do 3 times.

Make it easier: Hold the plank without shifting.

Up the challenge: Raise one foot off the floor and then shift.

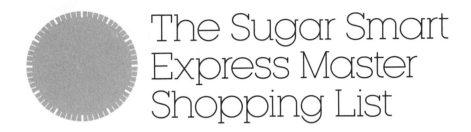

The Sugar Smart Express Master Shopping List

Although each meal and snack contains its own "shopping list," we've included this master list to make shopping a breeze. Make four copies of this list, one for each phase. As you begin each phase, choose the meals and snacks you want to eat. Then enter the quantities of the items you need, based on the meals and number of servings you're making. Make sure your pantry is fully stocked with the Flavor Boosters in Chapter 6.

CANNED FOODS	
__Beans, black	__Crab
__Beans, kidney	__Salmon
__Beans, pinto	__Sauerkraut, low-sodium
__Beans, white	__Tomatoes, diced
__Chickpeas	__Tuna, in oil

DAIRY	
__Butter, unsalted	__Cheese, Parmesan
__Cheese, Cheddar, shredded	__Cheese, ricotta, part-skim
__Cheese, Cheddar, sliced	__Cream cheese, reduced-fat
__Cheese, cottage, low-fat	__Milk, fat-free
__Cheese, feta	__Pudding, vanilla, low-fat
__Cheese, goat	__Yogurt, Greek, plain, 0%
__Cheese, mozzarella, part-skim	__Yogurt, plain, low-fat

(continued)

The Sugar Smart Express Master Shopping List (cont.)

FLAVOR BOOSTERS AND SWEET TREATS

__Apricots, dried, unsweetened
__Chips, chocolate, dark
__Cocoa powder, unsweetened
__Coconut, shredded, unsweetened
__Crackers, graham
__Cranberries, dried
__Enchilada sauce, no sugar added
　(such as Las Palmas brand)
__Fruit spread, 100% fruit strawberry

__Honey (local honey preferred)
__Hummus, prepared, any variety (such
　as Trader Joe's Organic Original
　Hummus and any flavor of Tribe or
　Cedar's All Natural)
__Marshmallows, regular
__Olives, Greek
__Salsa
__Syrup, maple, pure
__Wafers, vanilla

GRAINS AND BREADS*

*Buy only whole wheat or whole grain items; corn tortillas are permitted.

__Bread
__Bread crumbs (such as Ian's Whole
　Wheat Panko Bread Crumbs)
__Brown rice
__Buckwheat groats
__Bulgur
__Buns, hamburger
__Buns, hot dog
__Crispbreads (such as Wasa brand)
__English muffins (such as Thomas'
　100% Whole Wheat or Trader Joe's
　Whole Wheat British Muffins)
__Farro
__Oats, rolled

__Penne, whole grain
__Pitas (such as Ezekiel 4:9 Whole
　Grain Pocket Bread)
__Quinoa
__Rice, wild
__Tortillas, 6-inch diameter (such as
　Whole Foods 365 Organic Whole
　Wheat Tortillas or Food for Life
　Ezekiel 4:9 Sprouted Whole Grain
　Tortillas)
__Tortillas, 10-inch diameter (such as
　Food for Life Sprouted Corn Tortillas
　or La Tortilla Factory Sonoma Yellow
　Corn Organic Tortillas)
__Waffles, frozen

HERBS, FRESH*

*May use dried, if desired

__Basil
__Chives
__Garlic

__Ginger
__Mint
__Parsley

MEAT, POULTRY, AND VEGETABLE PROTEIN

__Bacon, center-cut
__Beef, ground, lean
__Beef, roast, lean, reduced-sodium
　(such as Boar's Head)
__Beef, sirloin, lean
__Chicken breast

__Eggs
__Egg whites
__Pork chop, bone-in
__Pork tenderloin, lean

__Sausage, chicken (such as Hormel
  Natural Choice Jalapeño Cheddar,
  Trader Joe's Spicy Italian, or
  Applegate Organics Fire Roasted
  Red Pepper)

__Sausage, turkey
__Turkey breast
__Turkey burgers, lean, 4-ounce patties

Vegetable protein

__Burger, veggie
__Edamame, frozen

__Tofu, extra-firm
__Tofu, soft

NUTS/SEEDS

__Almonds
__Butter, almond (such as Woodstock
  Farms, Maranatha, or Artisana)
__Butter, peanut, smooth (such as
  Smucker's, Santa Cruz, Maranatha,
  or Trader Joe's)
__Cashews, roasted

__Pecans
__Pistachios, roasted
__Seeds, chia
__Seeds, sesame
__Seeds, sunflower, dry roasted without
  salt
__Walnuts

PRODUCE

Fruits

__Apples
__Avocados
__Bananas
__Blueberries
__Grapes, red

__Kiwifruit
__Lemons
__Oranges
__Raspberries
__Strawberries

Vegetables

__Arugula
__Beans, green
__Bell pepper, red
__Bell pepper, yellow
__Broccoli, florets
__Broccoli, shredded
__Cabbage, purple
__Carrots
__Cauliflower
__Collard greens
__Corn (raw or frozen)
__Cucumber
__Eggplant
__Fennel
__Kale

__Lettuce, romaine
__Mushrooms, cremini
__Onions
__Potatoes, yellow
__Spinach
__Spinach, baby
__Tomatoes, grape
__Tomatoes, regular
__Tomatoes, sun-dried
__Zucchini

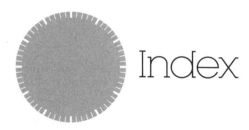

Index

Underscored page references indicate sidebars and tables. **Boldface** references indicate photographs.